keep
slim
exercises in
pictures

Margaret Ford

Ante-natal section by Erna Wright
Post-natal section by Mai Bryson

ILLUSTRATED BY BARRY FORSHAW

Wolfe

First published 1976
by Wolfe Publishing Ltd
10 Earlham Street
London WC2 9LP

ISBN 0 7234 0665 0

Printed photolitho by
Ebenezer Baylis & Son Limited
The Trinity Press
Worcester, and London

With grateful acknowledgements to:

Sally Denham,
The Bird Bath.

Iris Marsaglia and Sharon Lynn,
Westside Health Club.

John C. Langridge, MCSP, MSRG, SRP,
Medical Rehabilitation Centre, Camden.

A wide range of subjects is dealt with in picture-and-caption treatment in the Wolfe Pictorial Handbooks and the Wolfe Long Books

THE WOLFE PICTORIAL HANDBOOKS

O 7234 0463 1	First Aid in Pictures
O 7234 0695 2	Fruit and Vegetable Growing in Pictures
O 7234 0665 0	Keep Fit and Slimming Exercises in Pictures
O 7234 0642 1	Mending Things in Pictures
O 7234 0694 4	Motor Cycle Maintenance in Pictures

THE WOLFE LONG BOOKS

O 7234 0644 8	The Long Book of Car Maintenance
O 7234 0693 6	The Long Book of Cooking Skills
O 7234 0535 2	The Long Book of Horse and Pony Care
O 7234 0641 3	The Long Book of Match Fishing
O 7234 0653 7	The Long book of Coarse Fishing
O 7234 0654 5	The Long Book of Sea Fishing
O 7234 0587 5	The Long Book of Sewing in Pictures
O 7234 0545 X	Home Handyman in Pictures (in association with TV Times)

contents

Symbol key:
Easier exercises ★
Harder exercises ■

why exercise?

Medical evidence shows that we all need regular exercise. It not only keeps you fitter – it helps your looks. Shape is better when muscles are toned. Hair and skin are healthier when circulation is stimulated.

This is a 'dip-in and do-it' book for everyone. Shapers, revivers and relaxers are all planned with the help of experts – and tried out on dedicated non-exercisers to prove they are workable.

WHEN to exercise: There is no set time of day to exercise; do it when you feel freshest. It is not a good idea to jerk yourself awake or to go into action when you're tired. (The 'Jiffy liveners' have been specially planned for these times).

Leave exercising for at least an hour after meals. Otherwise, you're drawing blood to muscles that should be coping with digestion. Result: discomfort, indigestion.

A mammoth session every week will only leave you aching. Daily 'go's' get you trimmest, fittest. Ideally, make it the same time every day. It gets to be a habit that way.

HOW to exercise: You should exercise in the buff or wearing briefest light-weight clothes with plenty of give. The room should be cool – preferably not more than 70 degrees. Sweating gets your weight down, but only temporarily. Also if you're too uncomfortable you'll give up.

The right kind of pull. Whether standing, sitting or lying down to exercise, begin with a good stance. For this you will feel as if your head is being pulled up with a string from the crown.

HOW to choose. One look at the Contents and you'll know which section caters for you. Where appropriate, symbols have been used to tell you which are the harder, which are the easier exercises (* = harder; ■ = easier).

Easier exercises take longer to work, but unless you're really fit you'd be wise to start with them, or to begin your initial sessions with the body-suppling warm-ups.

You can swap exercises as much as you like – those featured individually. Limit your choice to no more than two for one area to begin with (except where there's a special routine). Keep exercise sessions down to 10–15 minutes for the first few days.

NOTE:
If you are receiving medical care – or have recently done so, you should not of course embark upon exercising without first referring to your doctor.

FOR WOMEN
warm-ups

These warm ups are undemanding movements which loosen up muscles for progressive exercises. Gymnasts use them to help save strain.

gentle stretch

1 Feet a little apart. Hands by sides.

2 Raise arms out and up above the head, breathing in for a slow count of five.

3 Lower arms back to sides and breathe out for a slow count of five.

take a breather

This is based on yoga.

1 Feet comfortably apart, arms at sides.

2 and 3 Raise arms out and up above head, breathing in.

4 Then, bending at the waist, fling arms down and forwards, expelling air in a hard gasp. Follow by three sharp out breaths.

Return to starting position. Do this three times only.

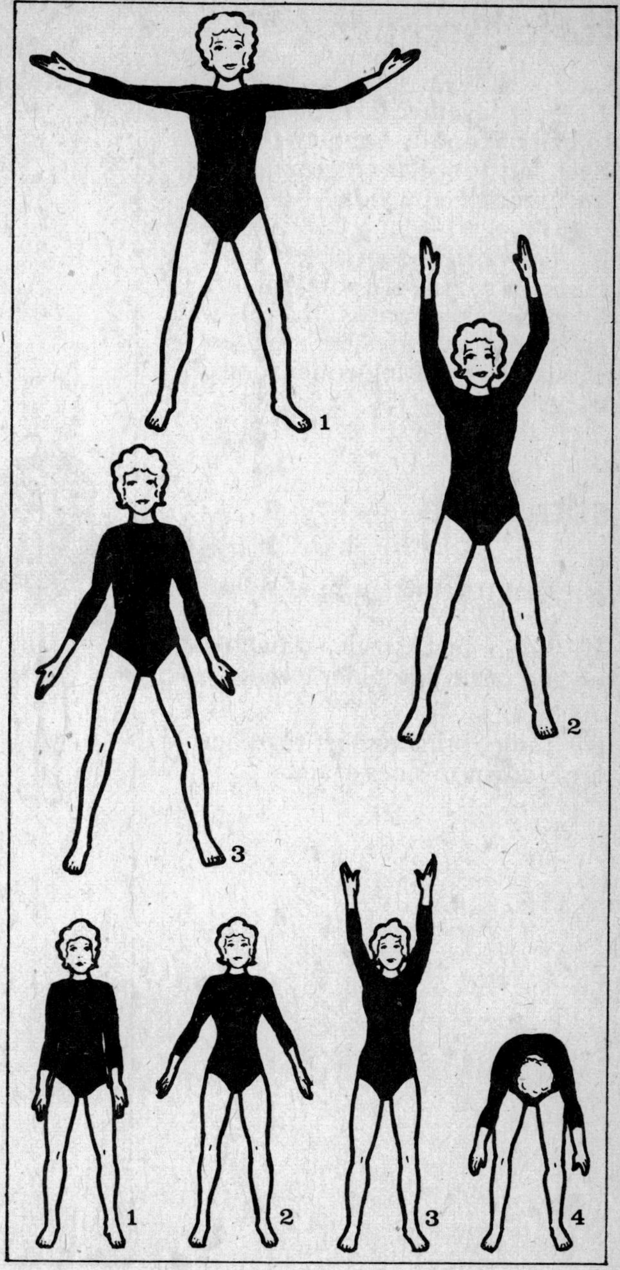

toffee stepper

1 Feet together. Lift right foot on to ball of foot by bending the knee. Keep left foot flat on ground. Pull thigh muscle upwards.

2 Lower right foot as left foot raises on to ball of foot. Pull left thigh muscle upwards. Jog this way briskly for two to three minutes without ever taking either foot off the ground.

star jump

1 Feet together, arms at sides.

2 Jump, feet astride, arms thrown up and out to shoulder level.

3 Jump, bringing feet together, arms down to sides again.

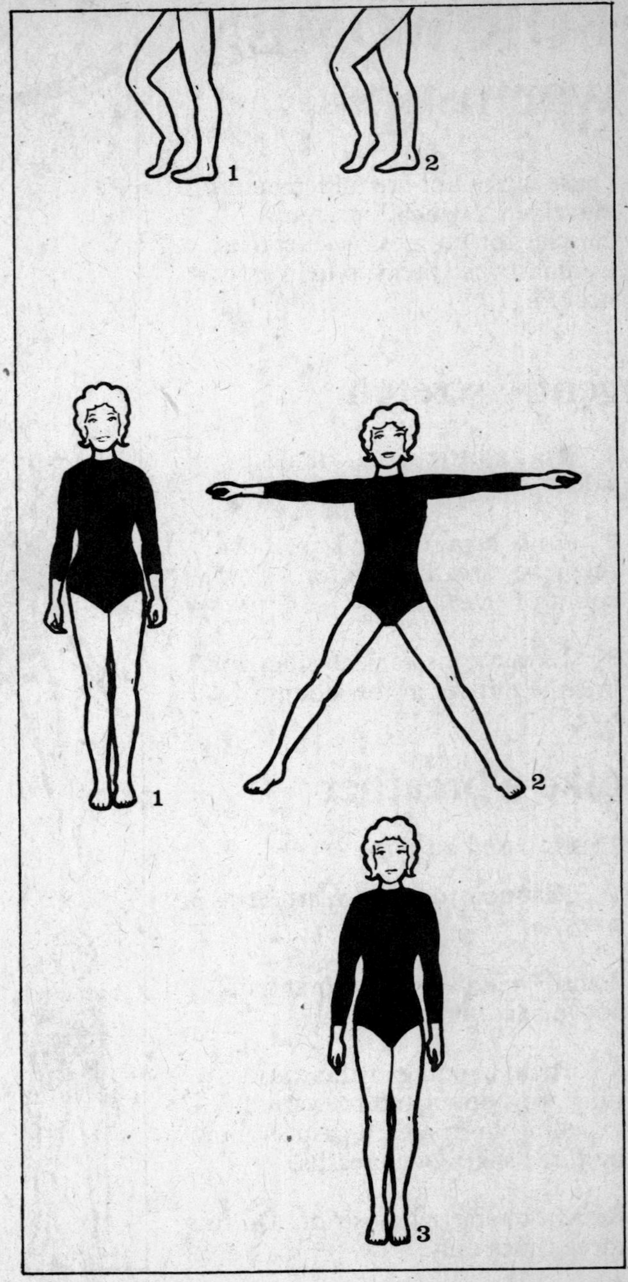

head turner

1 Feet comfortably apart. Hands on hips.

2 Keeping body still, circle head, dipping it as it comes forward.

3 Roll head back as you circle back.

4 and 5 Three circles clockwise, and three circles anti-clockwise.

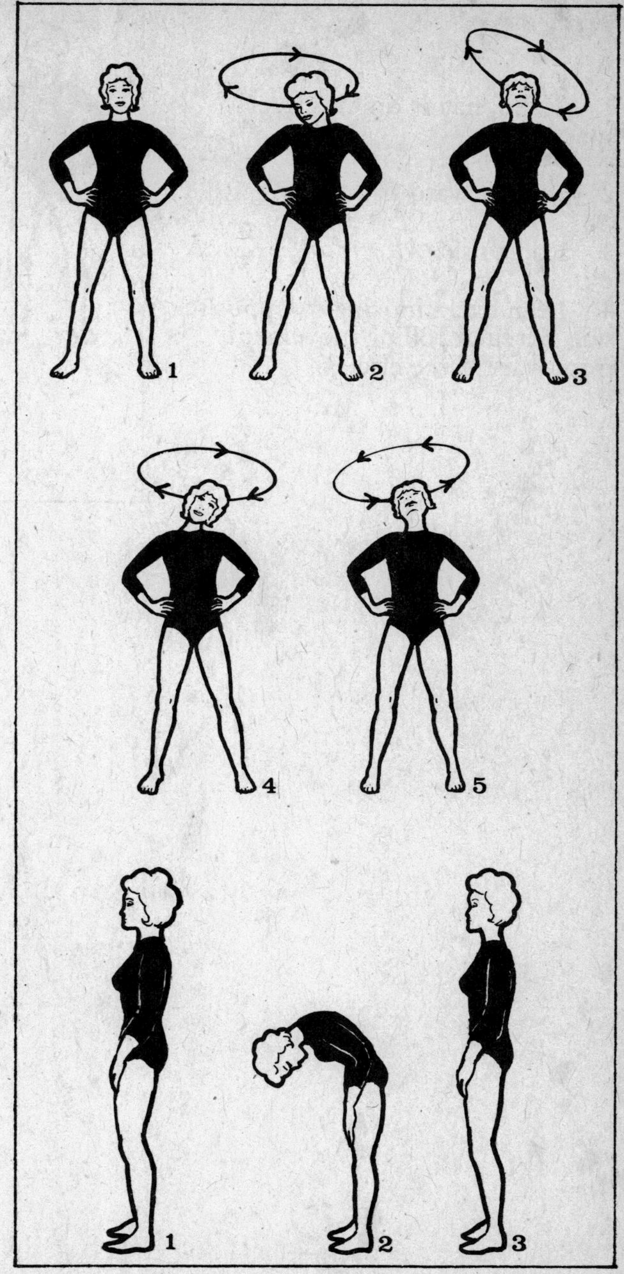

spine flexer

1 Stand feet together, arms down, hands on front of thighs.

2 Keeping hands well in, curve over to touch toes, vertebra by vertebra.

3 Straighten. Dip six times. Coil and uncoil *very* slowly.

roll top

1 Stand, hands on hips, feet apart.

2 Roll forward from hips.

3 Roll to side.

4 Lean back, moving to opposite side. Circular rolling movement from waist three circles.

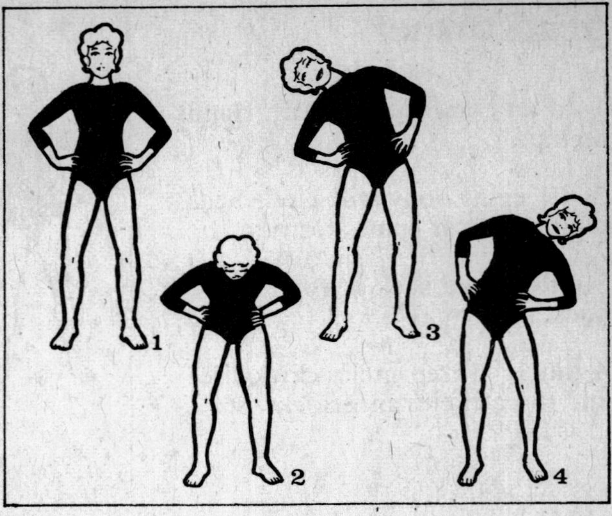

fat traps

These are the parts of you most likely to store fat. In women the main storage areas are stomach, seat and thighs; in men, the stomach. But you may have your own individual pockets and flabby muscle can make you look fatter than you are.

The exercises here are designed to go to work on podge wherever it plagues you. Of course, if you're generally overweight you need to cut your calorie intake too.

cuddle and fling

bust easy

1 Sit back on heels, back upright, arms at sides (Can be done sitting in a chair).

2 Lightly clench fists, bend elbows and bring arms up to shoulder level, closed palms facing body. Imagine you are cuddling a barrel.

3 Bounce shoulder blades together hard, pushing elbows back.

4 Fling arms across bust in a great hug – first right fist past left shoulder – left arm under and across.

5 Fling left fist past right shoulder, right arm under and across.

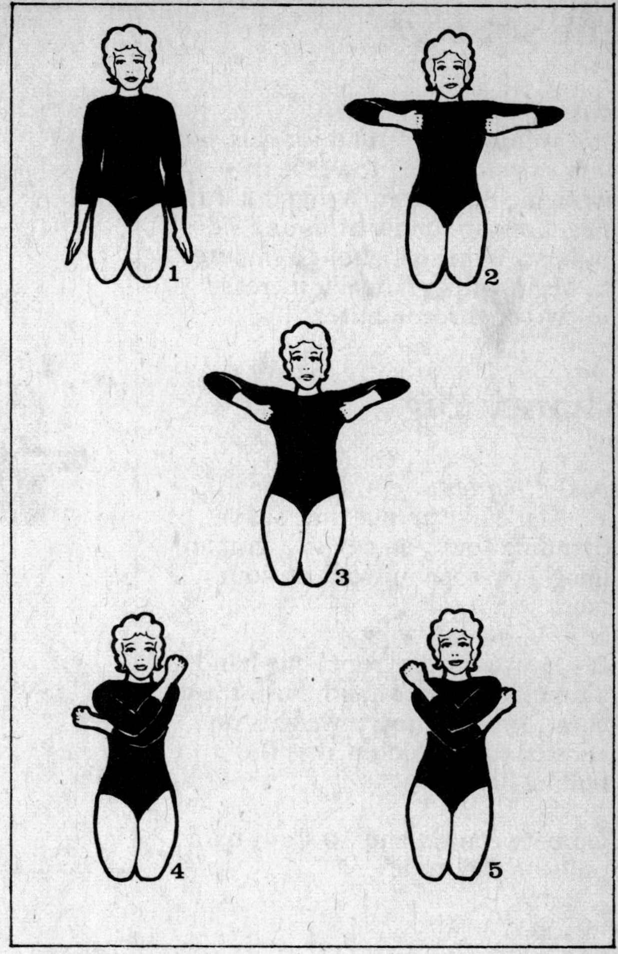

This exercise should be done very fast, with elbows up throughout, 10 to 15 times. Increase to two sets of 10, then two sets of 15, and finally two sets of 20.

the squeeze

bust easier
It's preferable to stand for this, but you can sit. Wring towel as if wringing out water. Wring it hard. Feel pressure under arms and sides of bust. Wring for about a minute to begin with, gradually increasing to two or three minutes.

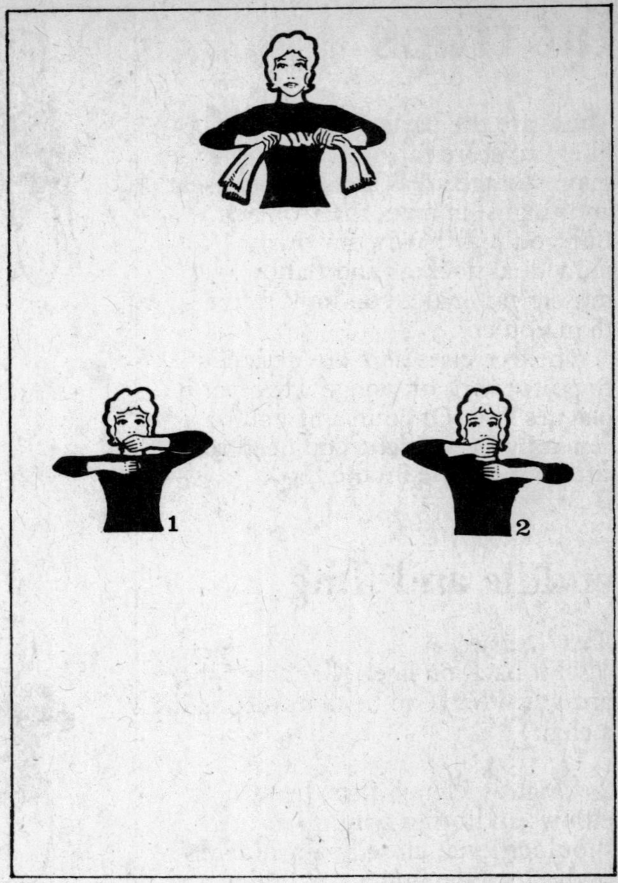

shanty tug

bust harder
1 Make like an old-time sailor. Standing (but you can sit), grip an imaginary rope in front of your face.

2 Heave on the 'rope' one hand at a time, hand over hand. Push from chest. Imagine heavy weights on ends of rope which makes the pulling harder.

Do between six and 10 slow, hard pulls on the 'rope'.

cross with a bounce

bust harder

1 Stand with feet comfortably apart, arms out at shoulder level, fingers stretched and palms facing forward.

2 Swing arms across chest, bouncing twice very firmly, trying to squeeze bust inwards. Keep elbows straight.

3 Swing arms out to sides again.

4 Drop arms firmly to sides, palms facing back.

Continued overleaf

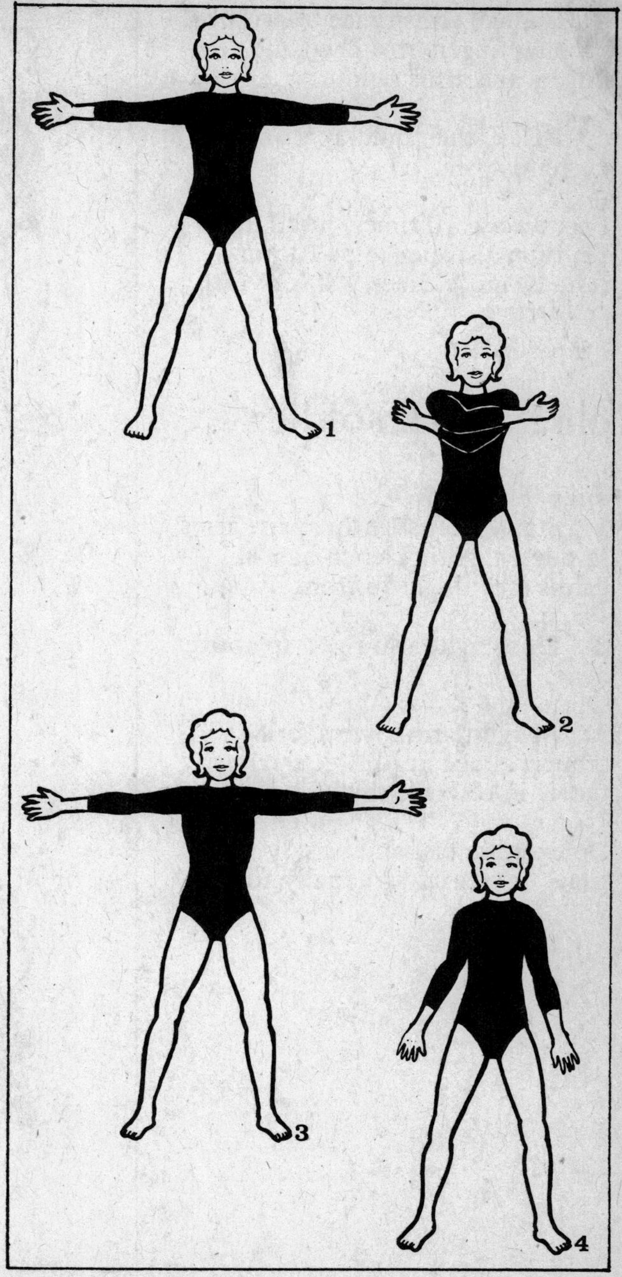

5 Bounce arms twice backwards, keeping fingers stretched and fingers and arms rigid.

6 Relax, then quickly go into exercise again.

Do exercise 10 times. Build up to 15, then a sequence of 10 times, rest, 10 more times. All very fast and strong.

clockwork soldier

midriff · easier

1 Stand, feet slightly apart, arms at sides. Lightly clench hands. Palms face thighs in front of you.

2 Raise right arm right up above head.

3 As right arm lowers, bring left arm up above head. Keep palms facing in towards thighs.

Do exercise fast and briskly 10 times, increasing gradually to 15.

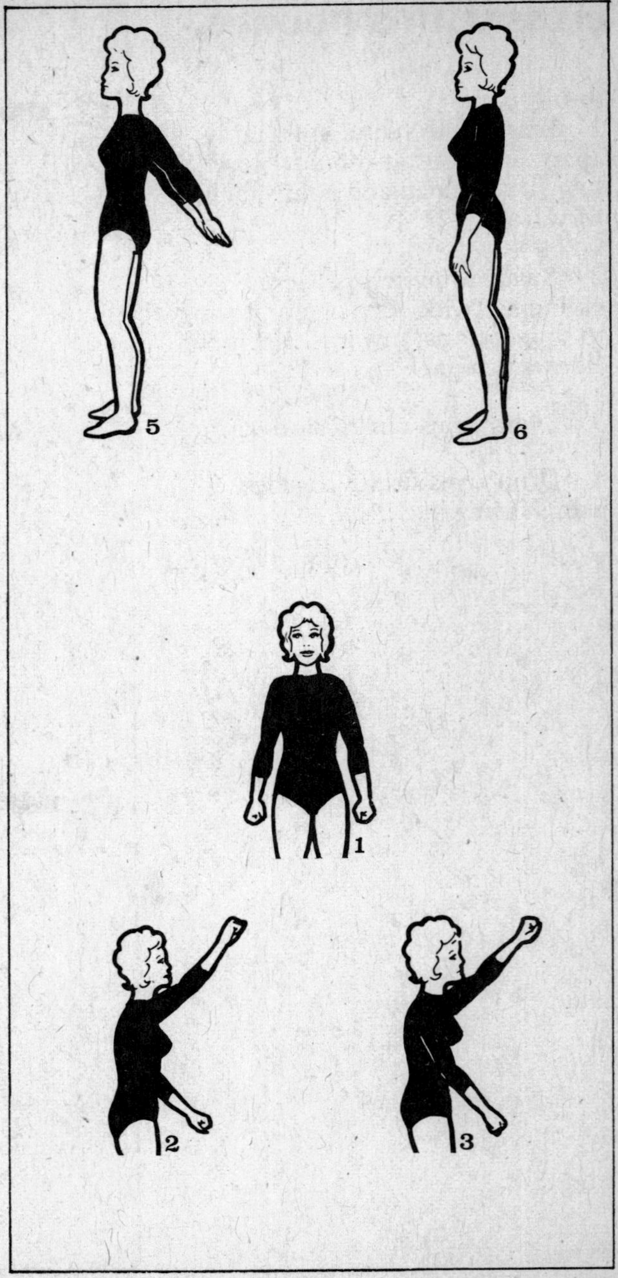

making arcs

midriff   easy

1   Lying, legs out straight, hold heavy book, or canned food, or any weight (three to five lbs) on thighs.

2 and 3   Lifting the weight, pull arms slowly and firmly up and back over head, keeping elbows straight.

4 and 5   Lower arms slowly until weight is once again resting on thighs.

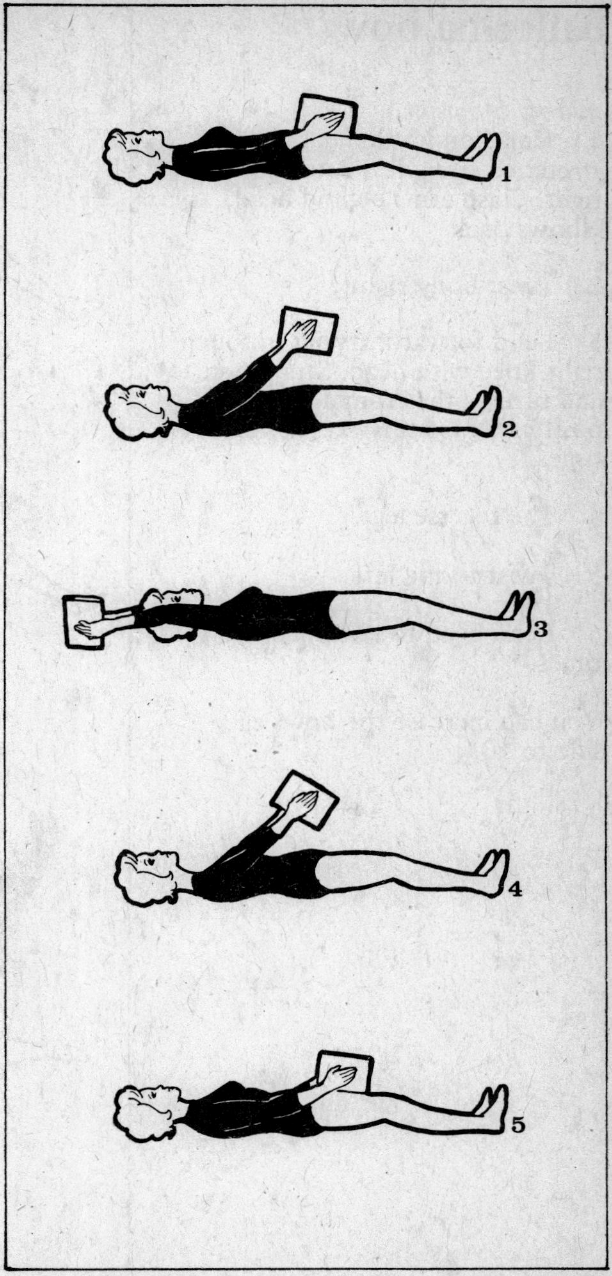

ballerina bow

midriff harder

1 Kneel on left knee, right leg stretched straight out towards right. Clasp arms behind head, elbows back.

2 Twist body right.

3 Bend forward, trying to touch right knee with head. Straighten and turn to the front again, as in position 1. Do this exercise five times.

4 The reverse legs.

5 Twist to the left.

6 Bend head to left knee five times.

You can increase the bows each side to 10.

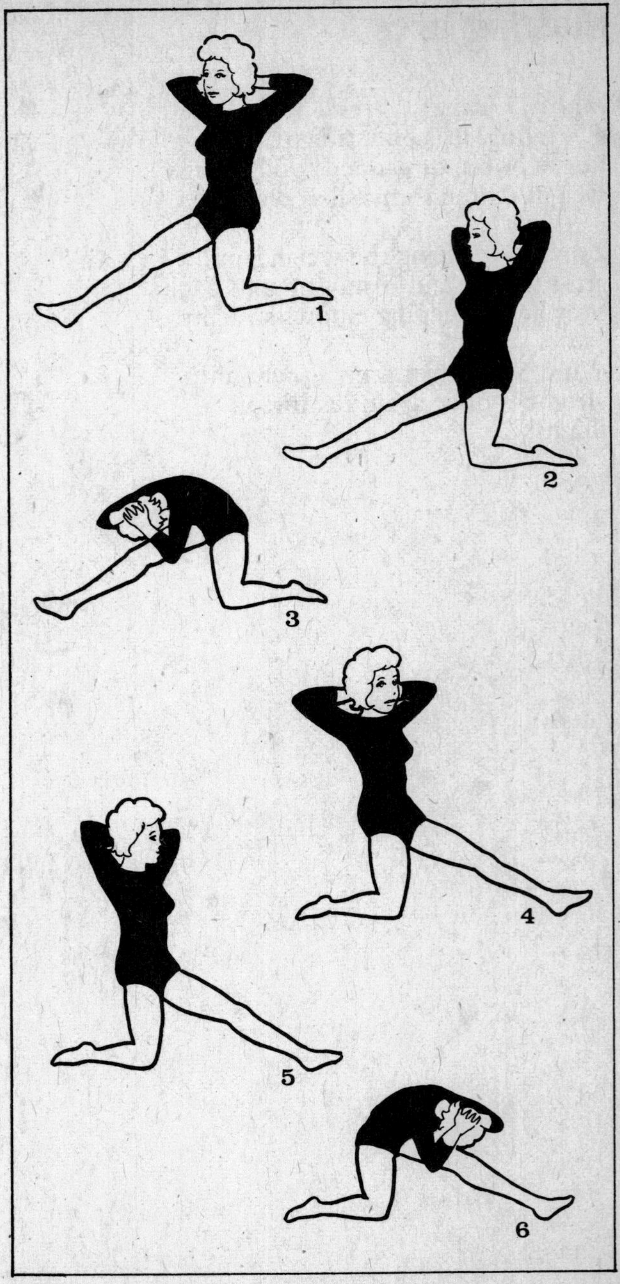

bell ringer

midriff   easier

1   Stand, feet about a foot apart, arms at sides.

2   Raise arms forward and right above head. Push up arms three or four times, trying to reach further with each push.

3   Drop arms down briskly to toes and bounce hands three times.

4   Then bounce hands to floor through legs, as far back as you can manage, three times.

5   Swing arms straight up again.

Do whole movement five times, working up to 15. Fast and vigorous.

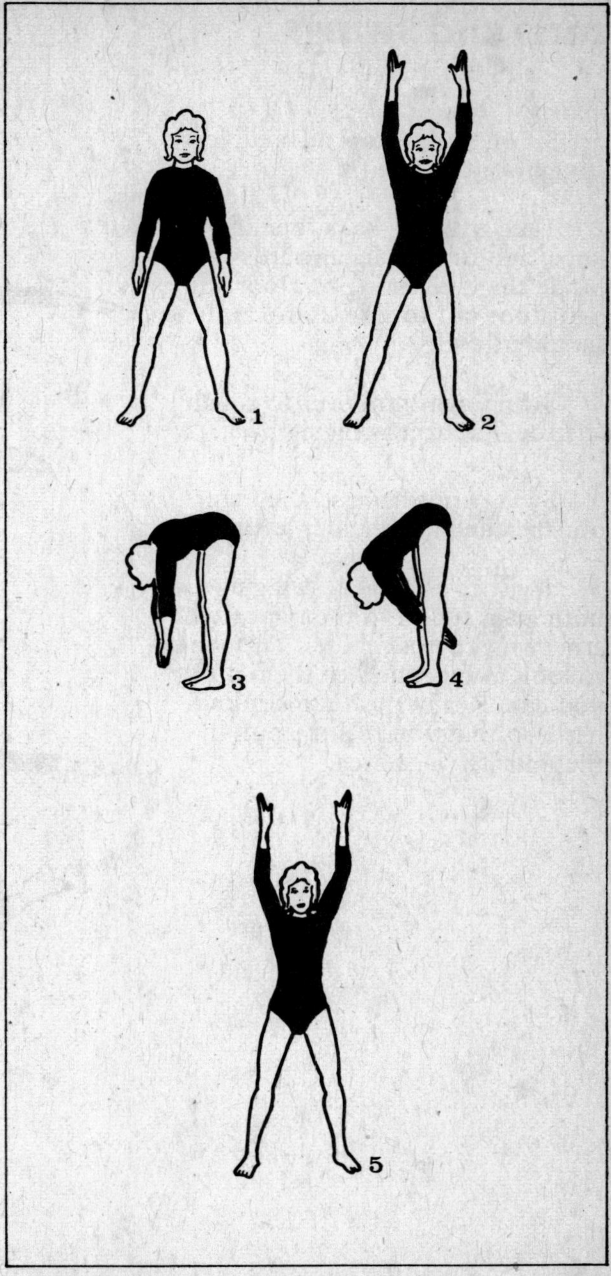

curls and swings

midriff harder
1 Sit on floor, arms relaxed, legs straight out in front.

2 Take right leg back, bending knee, and turning leg inwards so inside thigh is resting on floor and right foot out to side. Raise arms to shoulder level.

3 Swing right arm over to touch left toe, left arm swinging back.

4 Swing arms back so they are outstretched at shoulder level again.

5 Twist to the right, swinging both arms round to the right (left arm swings across chest). Turn head to look as far round to the right as you can. Really push arms round hard, so that you feel the pull in the midriff/waist area.

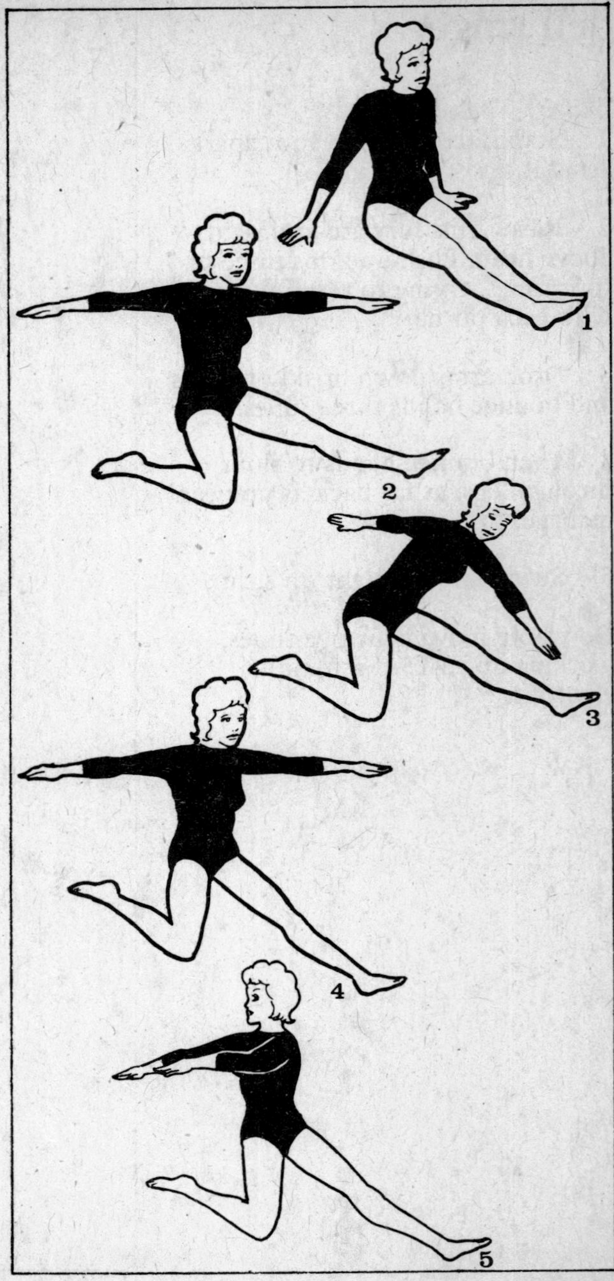

6 Swing arms back to stretch out sideways once more.

7 Bend left leg back, with right leg kept straight, and swing left arm to right toe.

8 Swing arms back to stretch out sideways.

9 Twist to left, arms out sideways again.

10 Relax, with legs straight out in front.

The exercise can be built up gradually to 15 times on each side.

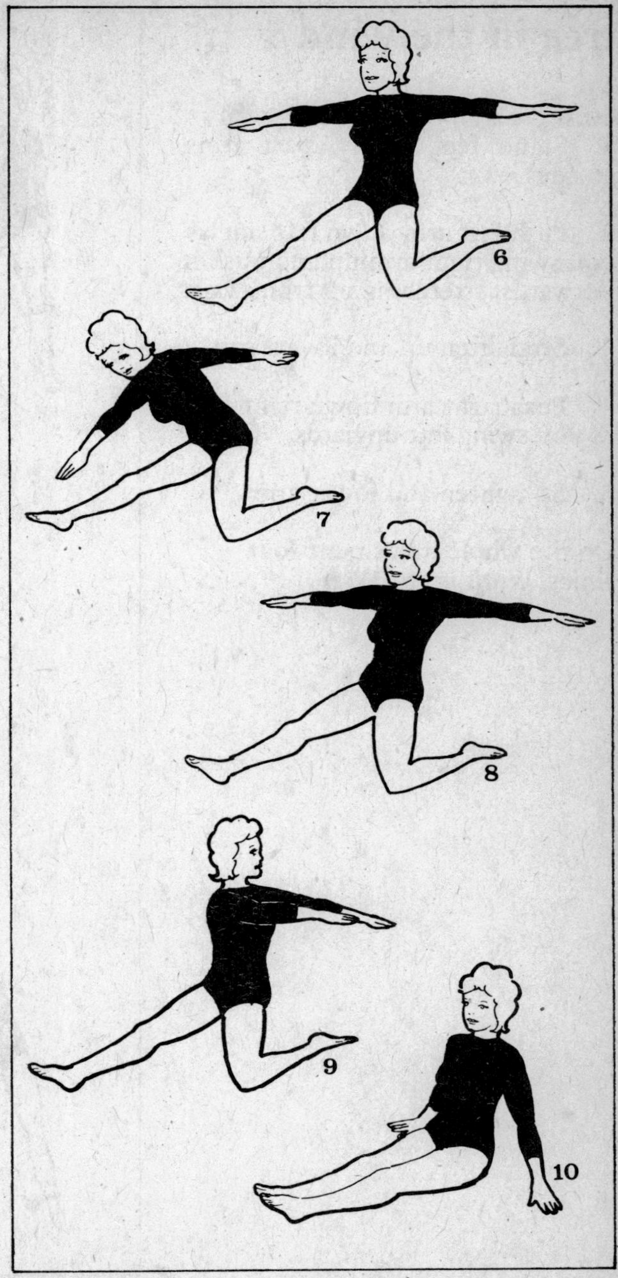

tree in the wind

waist easy

1 Stand, feet slightly apart, arms at sides.

2 Push left arm down left side as you swing right arm up and push it leftwards, stretching up from waist.

3 Straighten up and lower arm.

4 Push right arm down right side as you swing left upwards.

5 Straighten and lower arms.

Do the whole movement four times. Work up to 12.

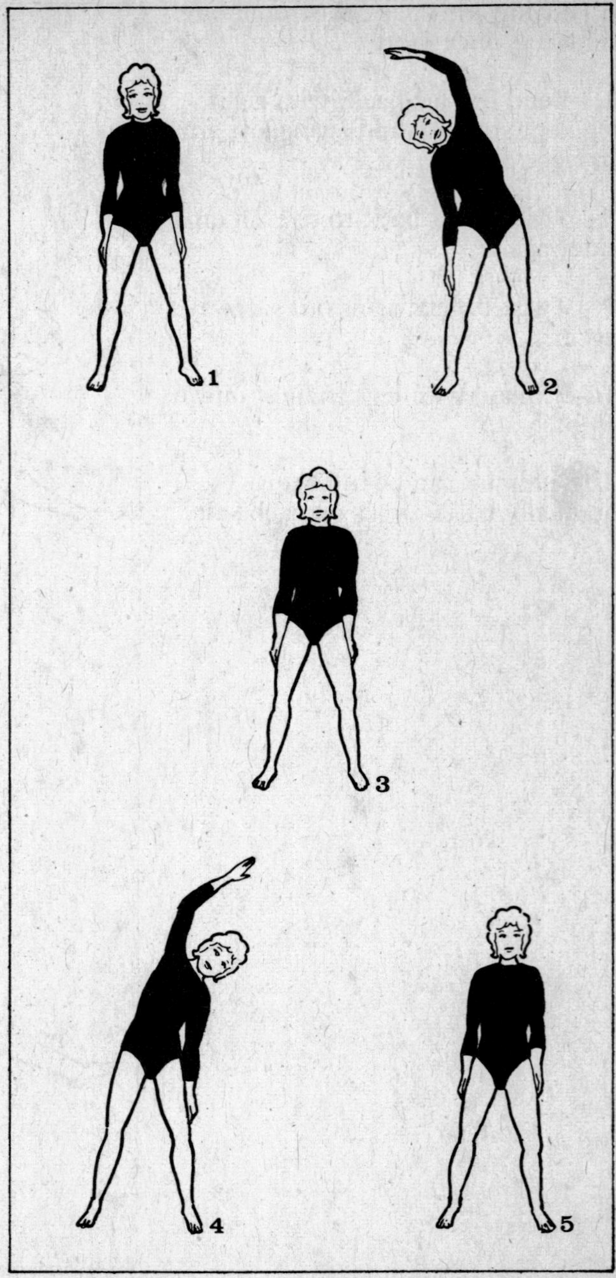

waist beano

waist *easier*

You need: a bean bag or an old sock filled with about 1 lb (can be less) of split peas, conkers or porridge oats. (Play safe and put them in an inner plastic bag.)

1 Feet together, bag in both hands, raise arms above head, keeping eyes on bag.

2 Drop bag behind you.

3 Squat on heels, knees apart, twist behind you to left to pick up bag. Drop it back in the same spot.

4 Twist behind to right to pick up bag.

5 Stand up again.

Do whole movement five to 10 times.

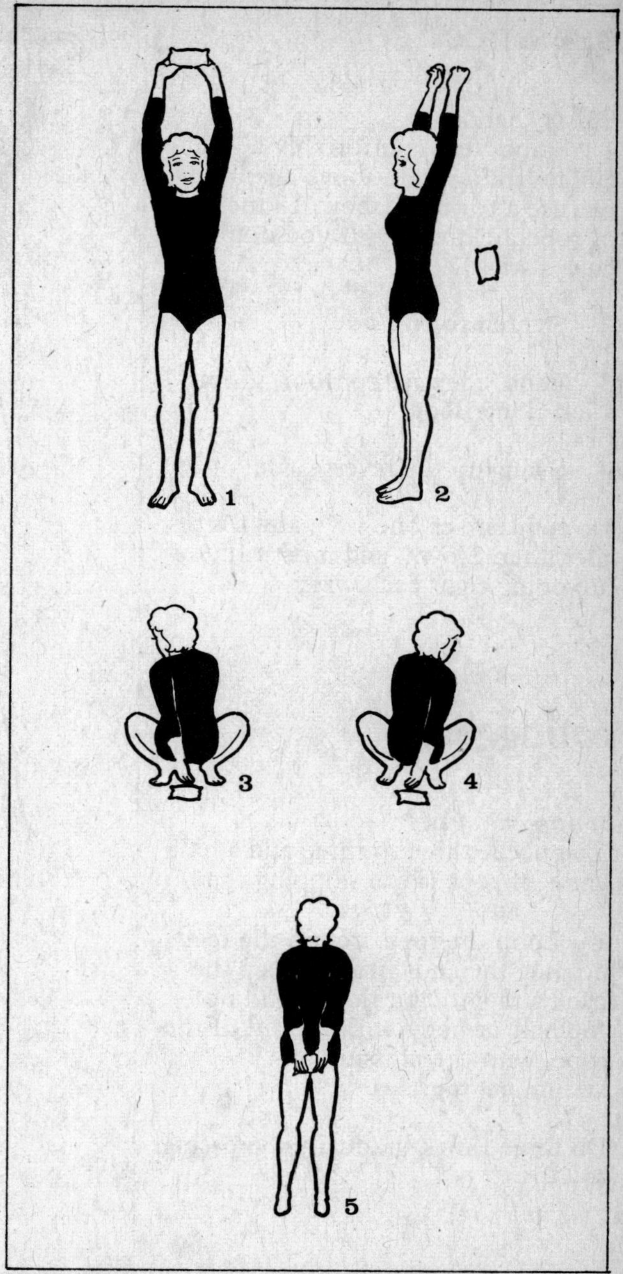

big wheel

waist   harder

1   Stand, feet comfortably apart. Hold walking stick above head (you can use a towel or about 18 inches of rope, held tautly, if you don't have a stick).

2   Stretch to one side.

3   Bend sideways to floor, sliding stick along floor.

4   Swing up the reverse side.

Do four circles one way, and four the other. Slowly add more till you are doing eight each way.

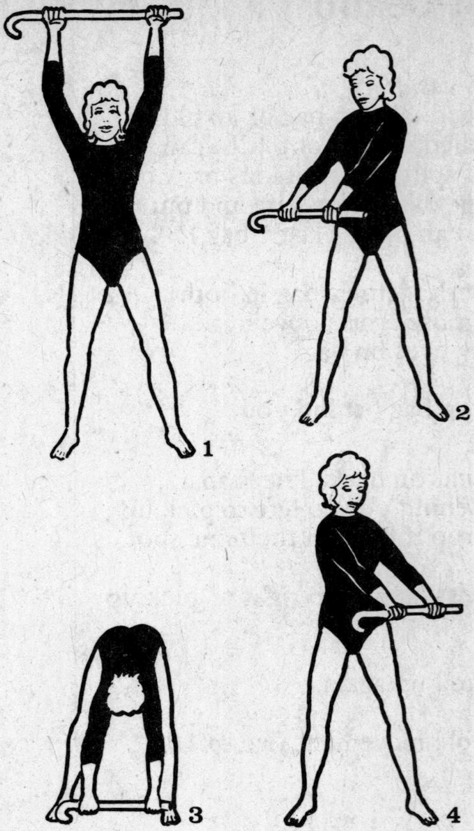

toboggan

abdomen   easier

You need: three to three and a half yards of rope (i.e. a skipping rope).

1   Loop the rope around the feet, holding the ends firmly. Keep the back straight, and slowly pull up top half of body with the aid of the rope, with the pressure on abdominal muscles.

Do three times, gradually increasing to 10.

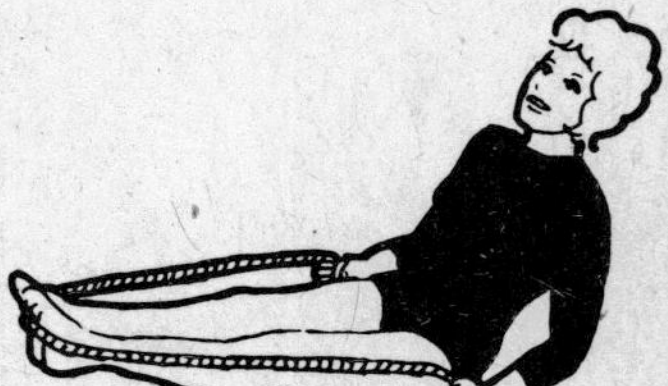

back down and leg lift

abdomen easy

1 Lie on floor, arms out at shoulder level. It is important, before you begin, to push the small of your back hard into the floor.

2 Raise right leg straight up in the air at an angle of 45 degrees. Hold for a slow count of three.

3 Lower right leg slowly.

4 Raise left leg.

Continued overleaf

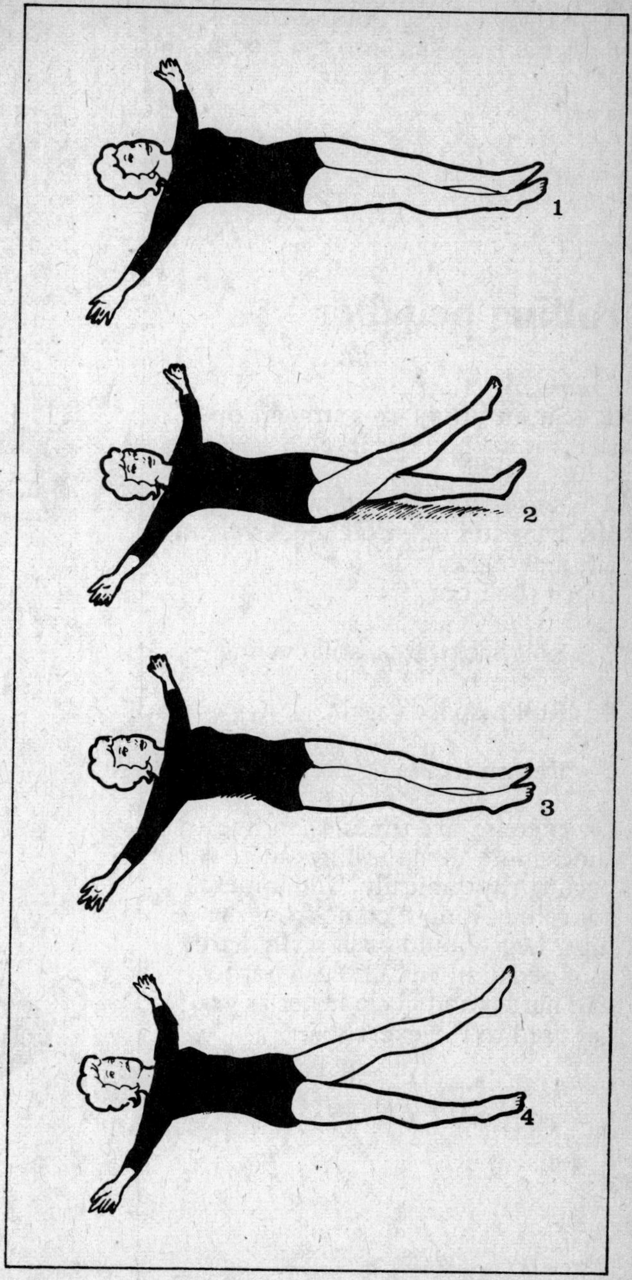

5 Lower left leg. All the time push the back flat into the floor.

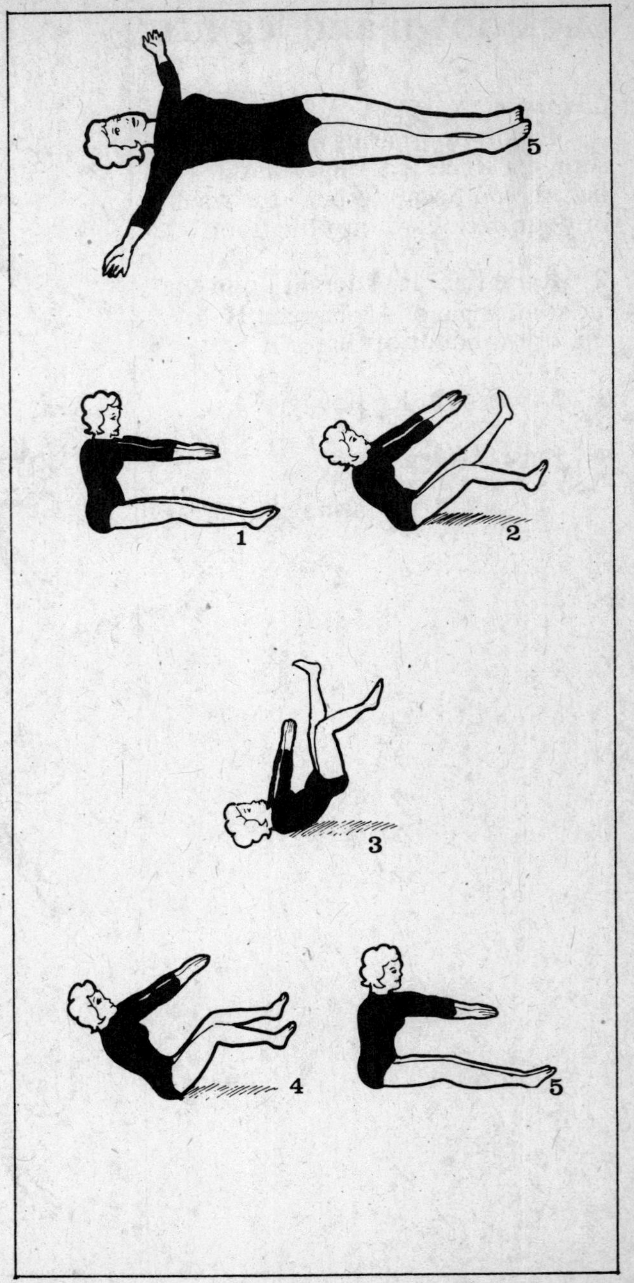

rolling pedaller

abdomen hard

1 Sit on floor, arms straight out in front at shoulder level.

2 Raise feet a little way into the air, arms still outstretched. Cycle in air, making sure the feet don't touch the floor.

3 Roll backwards, still cycling.

4 Roll forwards again.

5 Return to sitting position.

Do exercise five times, then five times more. Keep rolling and cycling rhythmically. The impetus for rolling should come from the hips. Legs should push really hard, as if pedalling uphill. Push harder and harder and cycle faster as you get used to the exercise.

scissors

abdomen harder

1 Sit on floor, with legs wide, arms out sideways.

2 Pull in stomach and raise legs as high as you can without toppling. Part them as wide as you can.

3 Close and open legs five times.

4 Lower legs, keeping back straight throughout.

When you can take it, try another set of five, building up to four to six sets of five.

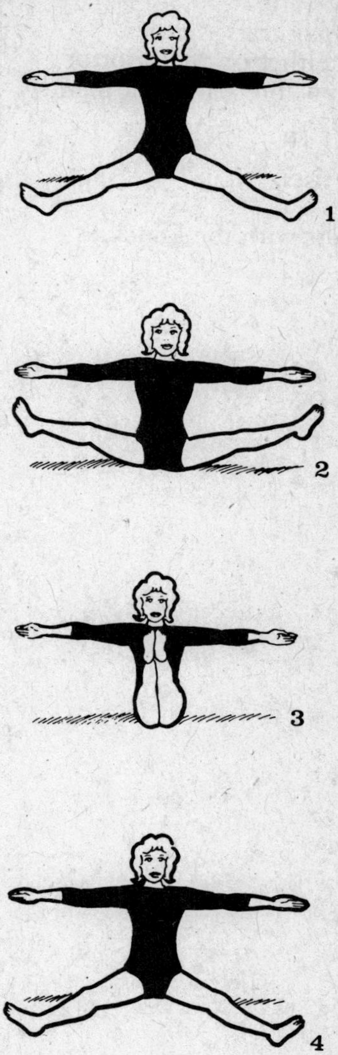

giant screw twist

backs of upper arms *easier*

1 Sitting, either on the floor or on a chair, put the arms out, palms up.

2 Clench fists.

3 Turn fists with the knuckles forwards.

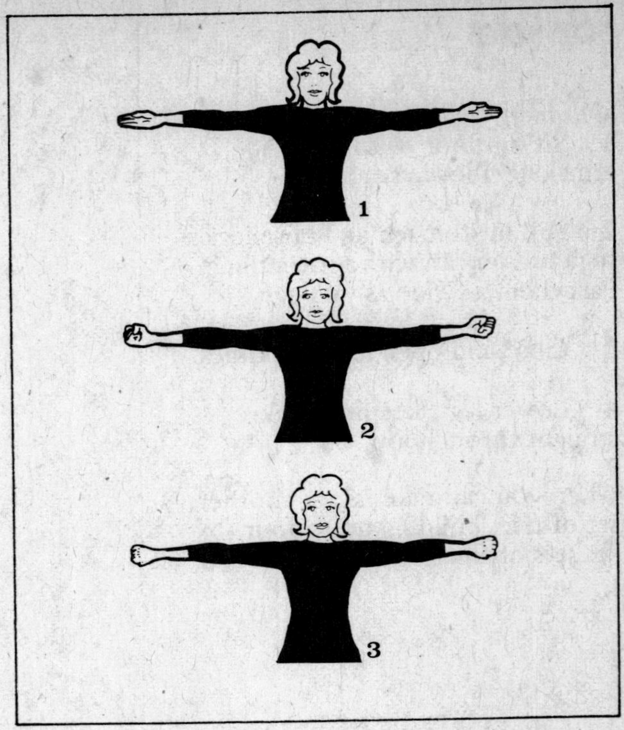

4 Open hands.

5 Twist hands further; so palms and elbows are upwards.

6 Twist back to original position.

This should be done very quickly. Really twist from the upper arms. Start with six full twists, increasing to 10.

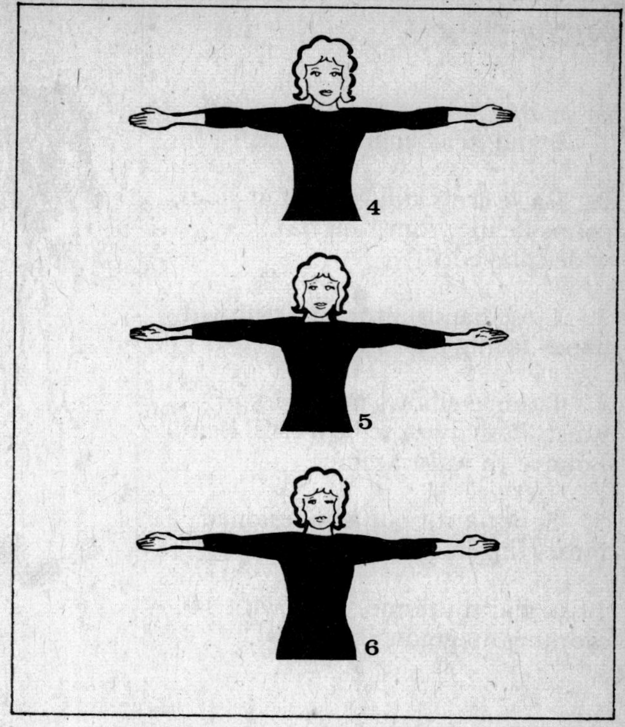

wing flex

backs of upper arms   *easy*

1 Stand, feet slightly apart.

2 Raise arms straight out at sides, palms facing front, fingers wide-splayed.

3 Close hands into fists, still with hands facing front.

4 Bounce elbows into sides of waist. Push away, elbows still bent. Bounce to waist again.

5 Shoot arms out at sides once more, fingers splayed.

Brisk and rhythmic. Start with 10, working up gradually to 30.

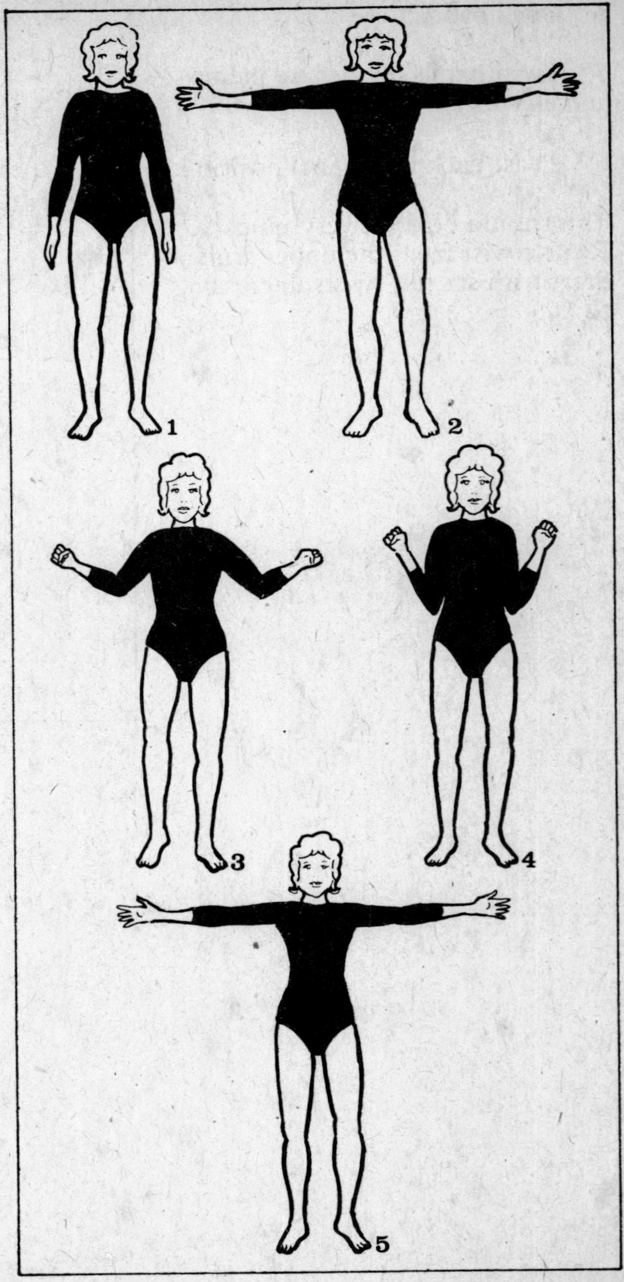

throw over

backs of upper arms *hard*

1 Standing, raise a 3 lb weight or can above the head. Keep the back straight, and side of arm and elbow close to head.

2 Bend elbow and lower the weight backwards to touch the back of shoulder.

3 Raise arm back above head again.

Very slow and deliberate. Ten times each arm, increasing, one at a time, to 15 or 20.

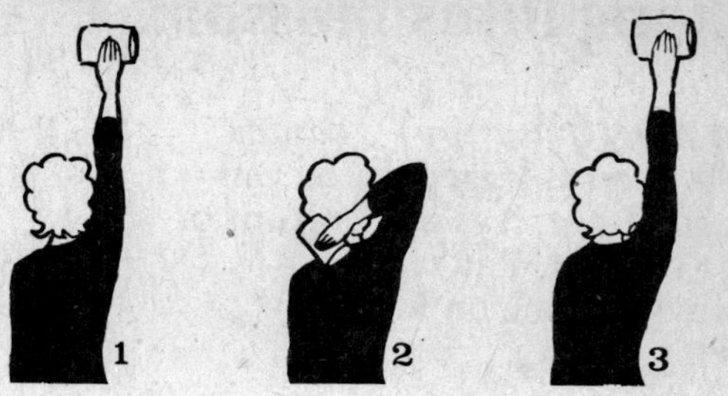

chop chop

front of upper arms *easy*

1 Stand with arms straight at sides, with 3 lb weight in right hand.

2 Bend right elbow, and slowly raise weight until it touches front of right shoulder.

3 Lower right arm to side slowly.

4 Transfer weight to left hand, and stand with arms straight.

5 Bend left elbow, and slowly raise weight until it touches front of left shoulder.

6 Lower left arm to side slowly.

Do this for 10 times on each arm, gradually increasing to 25.

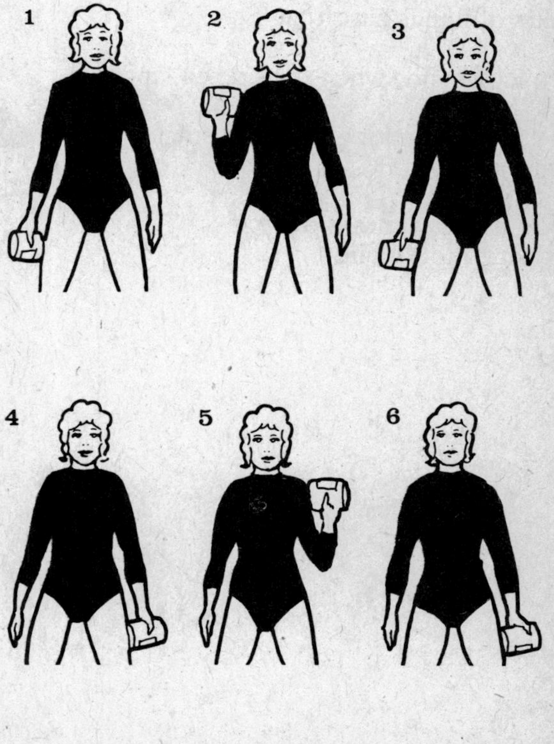

budding lotus blossom

upper arms (bust, too)   harder

1 Sit – cross-legged if you can manage, if not, legs out in front or sitting in chair. Put arms out sideways, resting on knees if cross-legged.

2 Breathe in as you bring arms out sideways and join hands together above head.

3 Breathe out slowly as you bend elbows and bring 'prayer' hands down in front of body, with the heels of hands hard together.

4 Part hands when they reach lap.

5 Start breathing in and raising arms again.

Do this five times, slowly in a flowing movement.

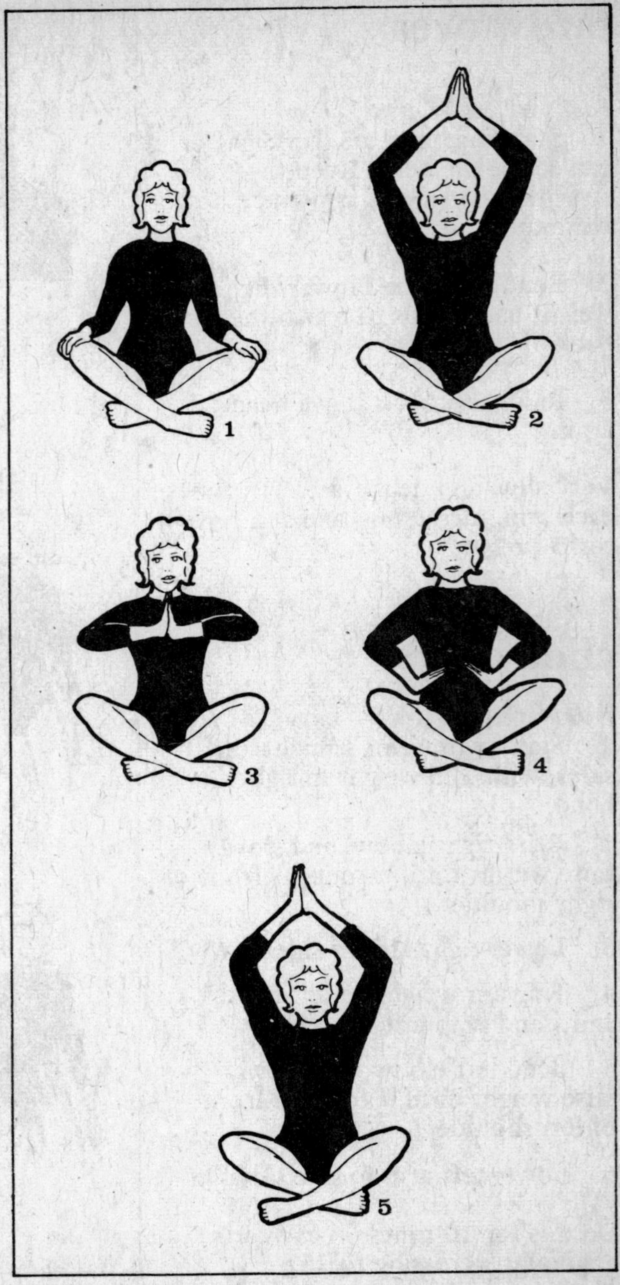

base bounce

seat easy

1 Sit, with legs out in front, straight and together, hands behind for support.

2 Bend right knee and place right foot by left calf.

3 Turn left foot towards floor. Using right foot as lever and taking weight on hands, lift seat and bounce on outside of left buttock twice.

4 Return to legs straight out position.

5 Bend left knee and place left foot by right calf. Turn right foot towards floor.

6 Return right foot to toes-up position and bounce twice on outside of right buttock.

Do the exercise fast and briskly 10 times, working up gradually to 20 times.

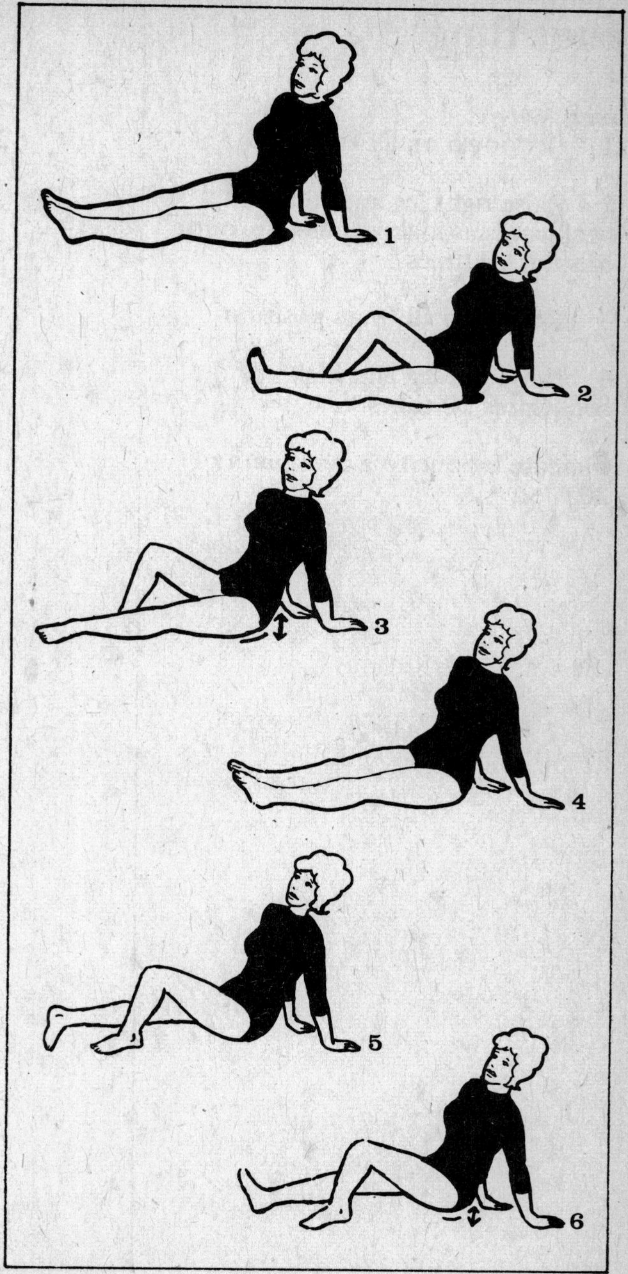

foot fling

seat easy

1 Get down on all fours.

2 Raise right leg and kick up backwards as high as possible, quite briskly, 10 times.

3 Return to all fours position.

4 Raise left leg and kick up backwards 10 times.

Increase by one to a maximum of 20.

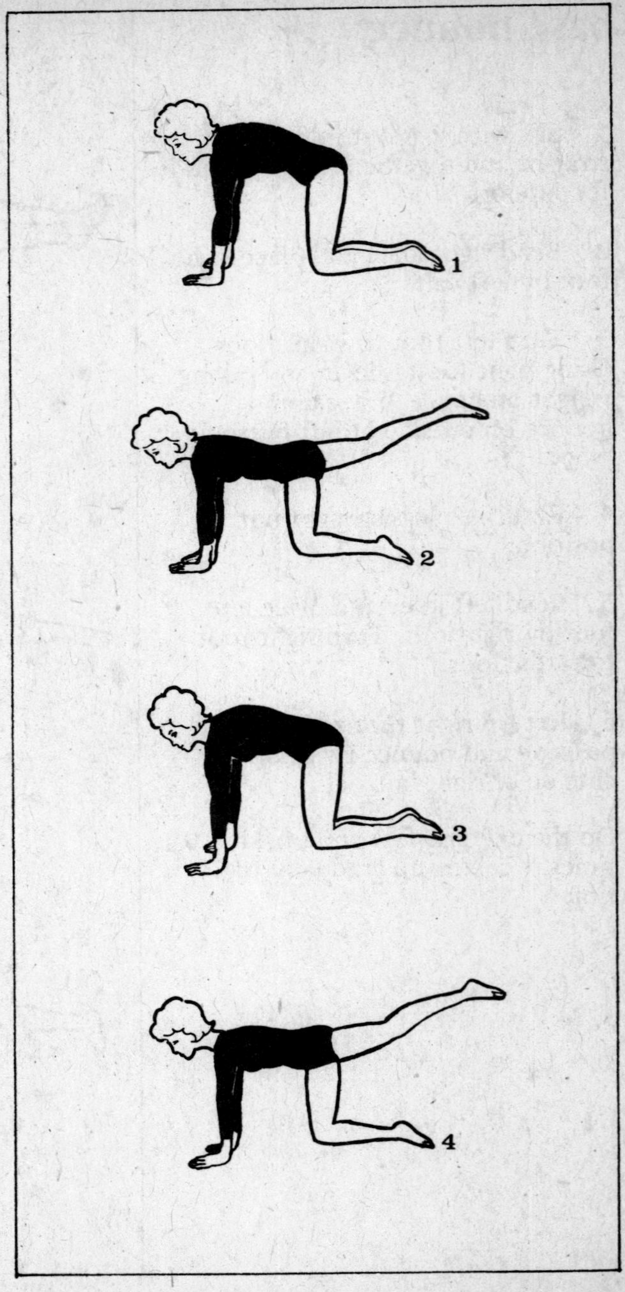

crossing toner

seat easy

1 Lie on stomach, resting head on hands.

2 Raise right leg straight up backwards in the air.

3 Cross it over left leg and touch floor with right toe on left side.

4 Raise right leg up again and lower back to starting position.

5 Lower right leg to floor.

6 Raise left leg straight up backwards.

Continued overleaf

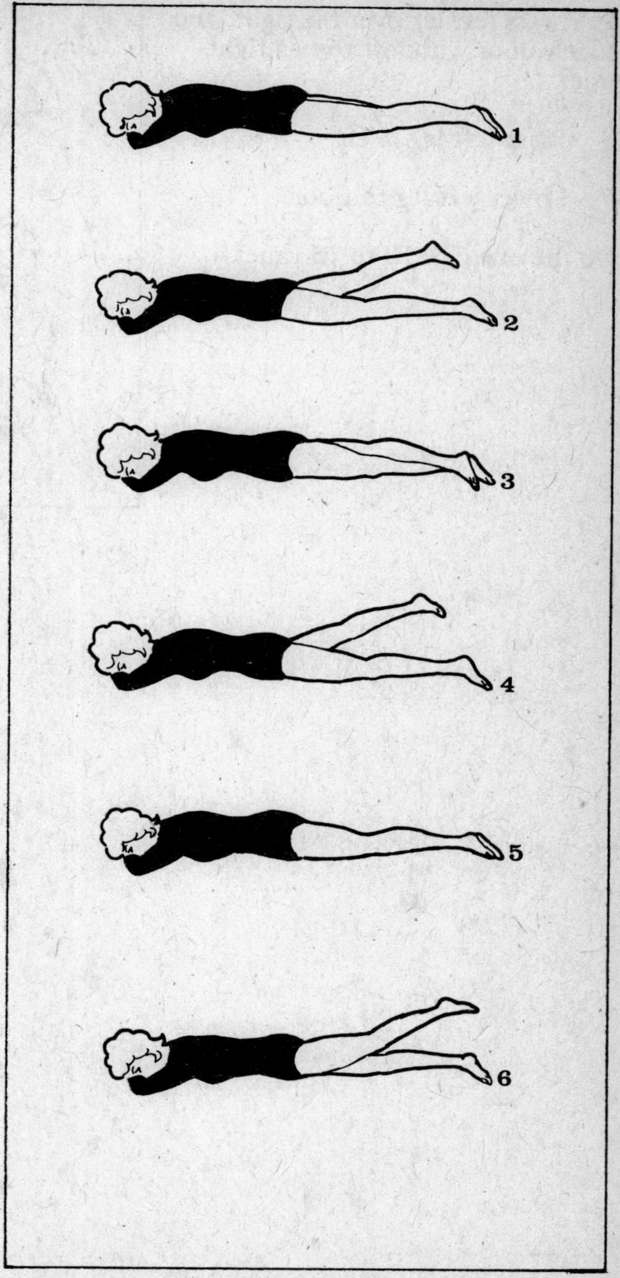

7 Cross left leg over the right, and touch floor with left toe on right side.

8 Raise left leg in air.

9 Lower left leg to floor.

Do the exercise 10 to 15 times.

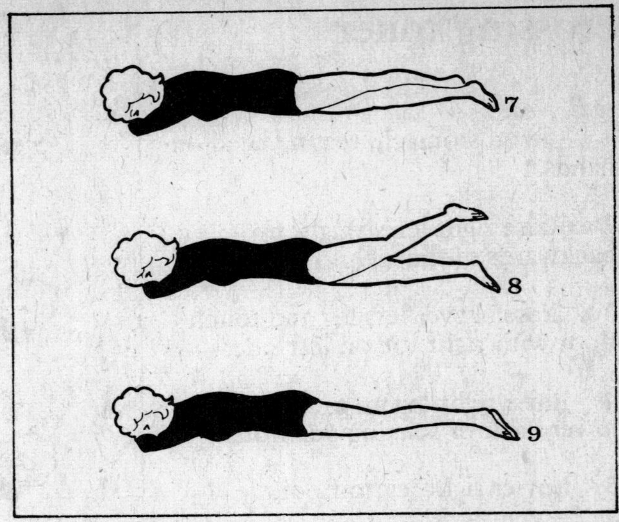

back and away

seat harder

1 Kneel on floor.

2 Bend forward and rest forearms on floor, elbows bent, palms down. Rest forehead on wrists. Raise right leg back and up, keeping knee very slightly bent.

3 Lower right leg.

4 Raise left leg back and up, keeping knee very slightly bent.

5 Lower left leg.

Do the exercise very slowly, keeping the back straight. Do five times for each leg, increasing gradually to 10.

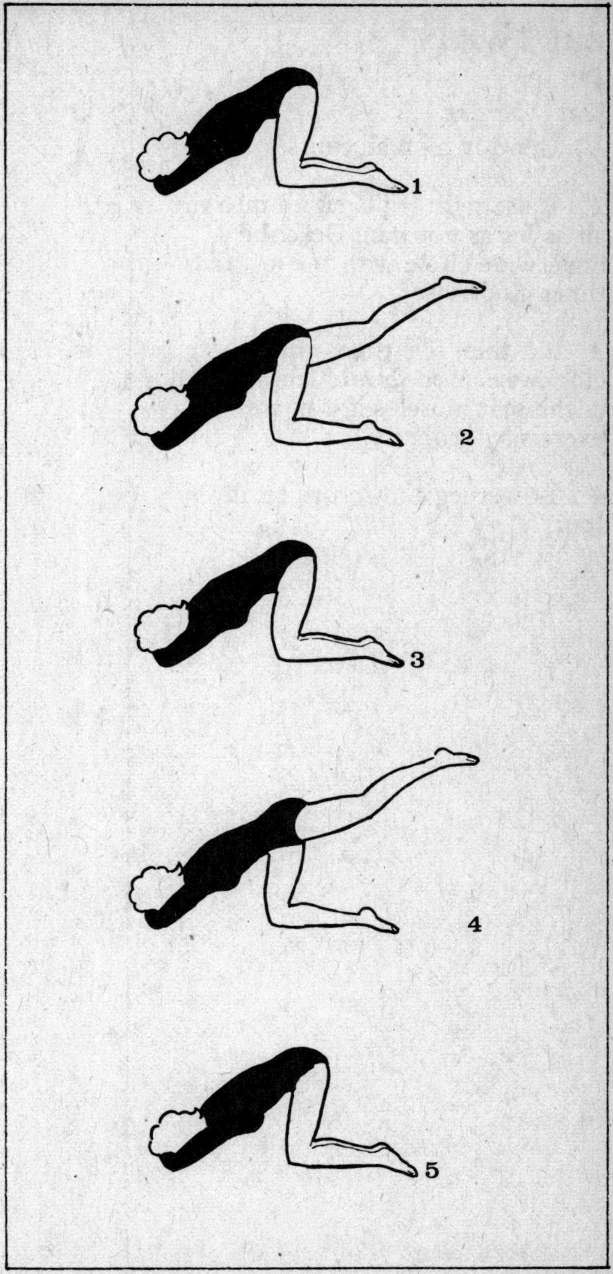

cat twirls

seat harder

1 Get down on all fours.

2 Raise right leg back up into the air as far as you can. Describe a high, wide circle with the leg, five times clockwise . . .

3 . . . then five times anti-clockwise. You should feel the pull in the seat muscles if you are exercising properly.

4 Lower leg and return to all fours.

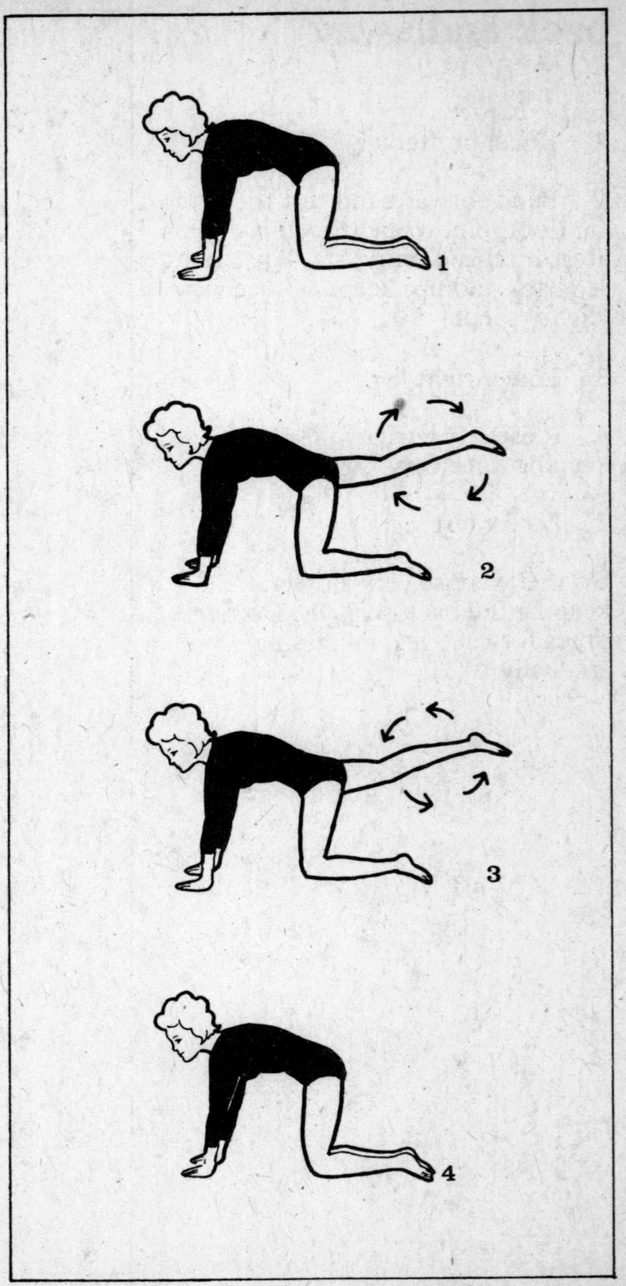

5 Raise left leg back up into the air as far as you can. Turn this leg in a high, wide circle, five times clockwise . . .

6 . . . then five times anti-clockwise.

7 Lower leg and return to all fours.

Gradually add one turn to each set of five up to a maximum of 15.

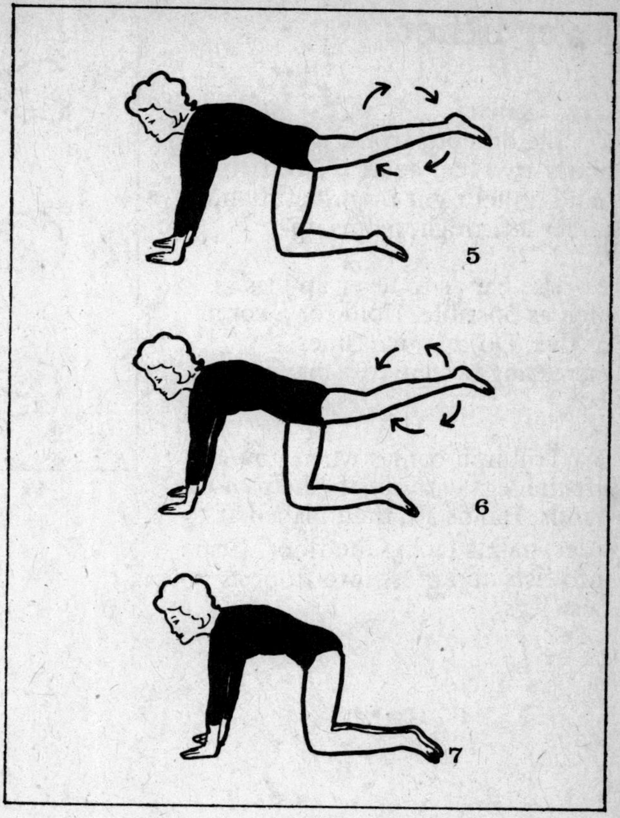

lever lither

seat harder

1 Lie on your front, with legs about two feet apart. Place right hand under right thigh, left hand under left thigh, palms up.

2 Use hands to lever up legs as high as possible. Hold for a count of five. Do this five times, increasing by one to a maximum of 10.

3 Triumph comes when you can lift the legs without the help of the hands. Hands are then placed at sides, palms facing the floor. Grip into fists and press into floor as you raise legs.

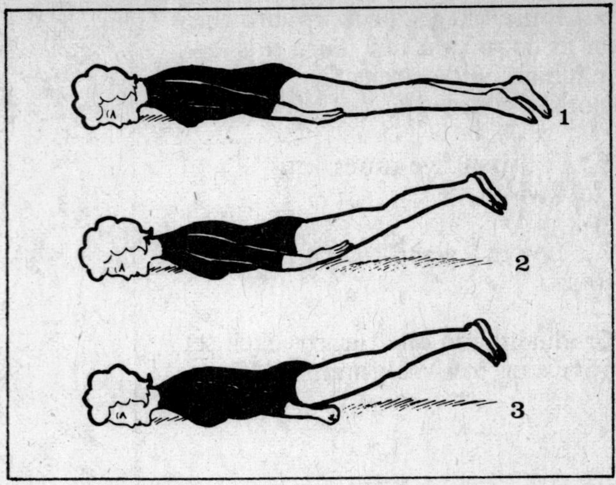

swinging arcs

backs of thighs and seat   *easier*

1 Stand, press hands on wall, arms at shoulder level, elbows slightly bent. Bend right knee and raise, trying to touch chest.

2 Kick back smartly, leg straightening.

3 Swing in to chest again.

4 Kick back.

5 Lower leg and repeat exercise with left leg.

Repeat movement 10 times, keeping a swinging rhythm. Try to avoid leaning forward as you kick leg behind.

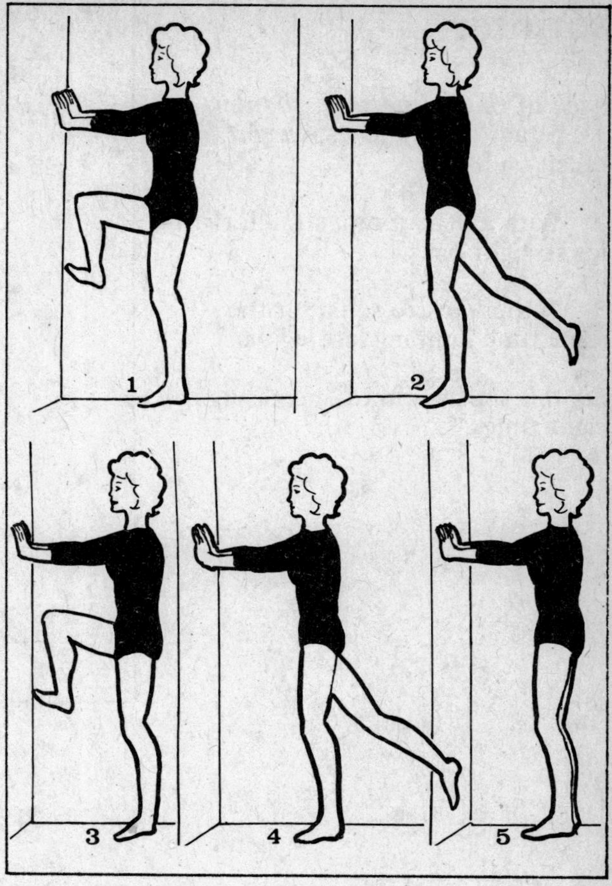

sprinter

back of thighs and seat *harder*

1 Squat on haunches, weight taken on hands.

2 With a little jump, stretch right leg straight back.

3 Jump back to squat, at the same time jumping left leg back.

Do this set five times, increasing to eight times.

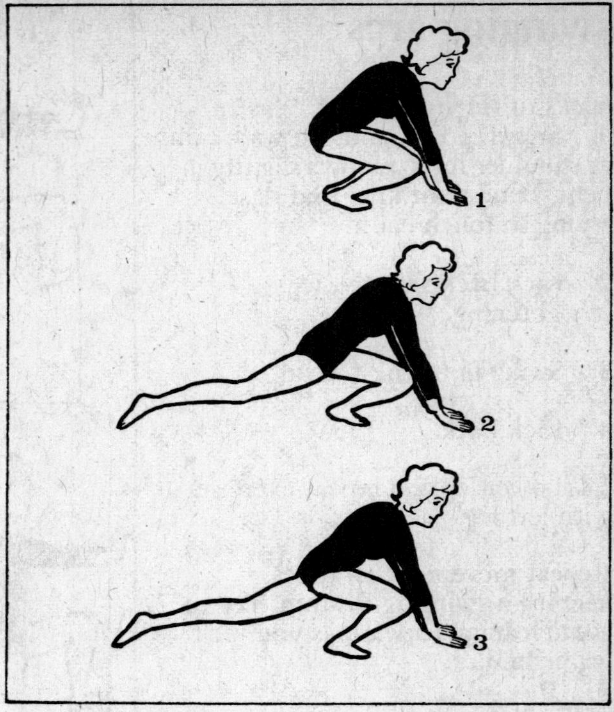

bus hopper

front of thighs *easy*

1 Stand in front of a well-supported low stool, or at base of stairs.

2 Step up on to stool/stair with right leg.

3 Step up with left, so both feet are up there.

4 Stand down with right foot.

5 Step down with left, so both feet are down again together.

The effect comes with doing the exercise quickly. Start with 15 times, then add another five, and five more as the legs become accustomed to it.

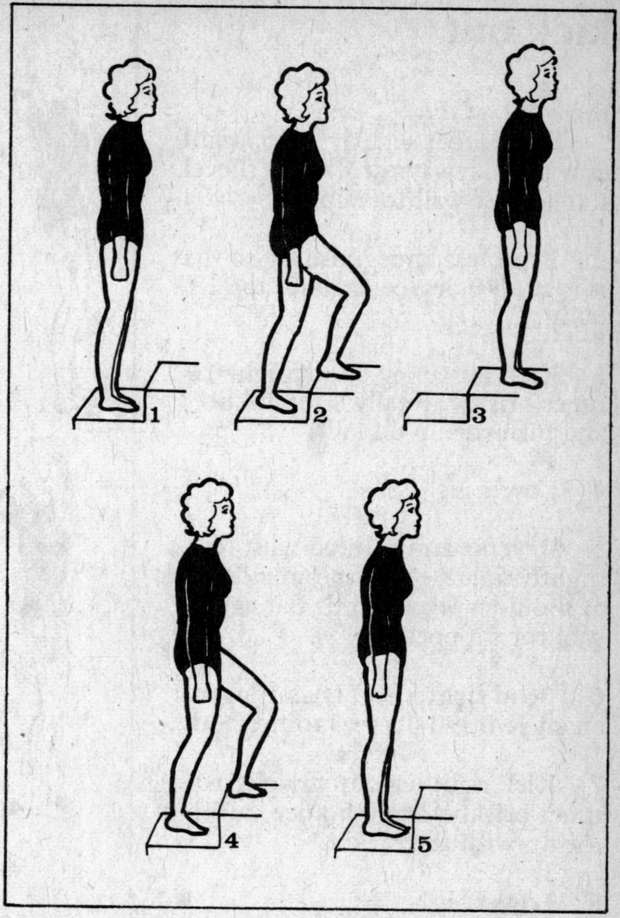

kick out

for front of thigh *easy*

1 Stand, feet slightly apart, right arm out sideways at shoulder level, flat against wall for support.

2 Bend left knee, raise leg so that it is at a 90 degree angle to the body.

3 Kick raised leg out straight 10 times briskly. Really stretch knee and turn toe up on kick.

4 Lower leg.

5 Reverse arms. Stand with feet slightly apart, left arm out sideways at shoulder level, hands flat against wall for support.

6 Bend right knee, raising leg at an angle of 90 degrees to the body.

7 Kick right leg out straight 10 times briskly. Stretch knee, turning toe up with the kick.

8 Lower leg.

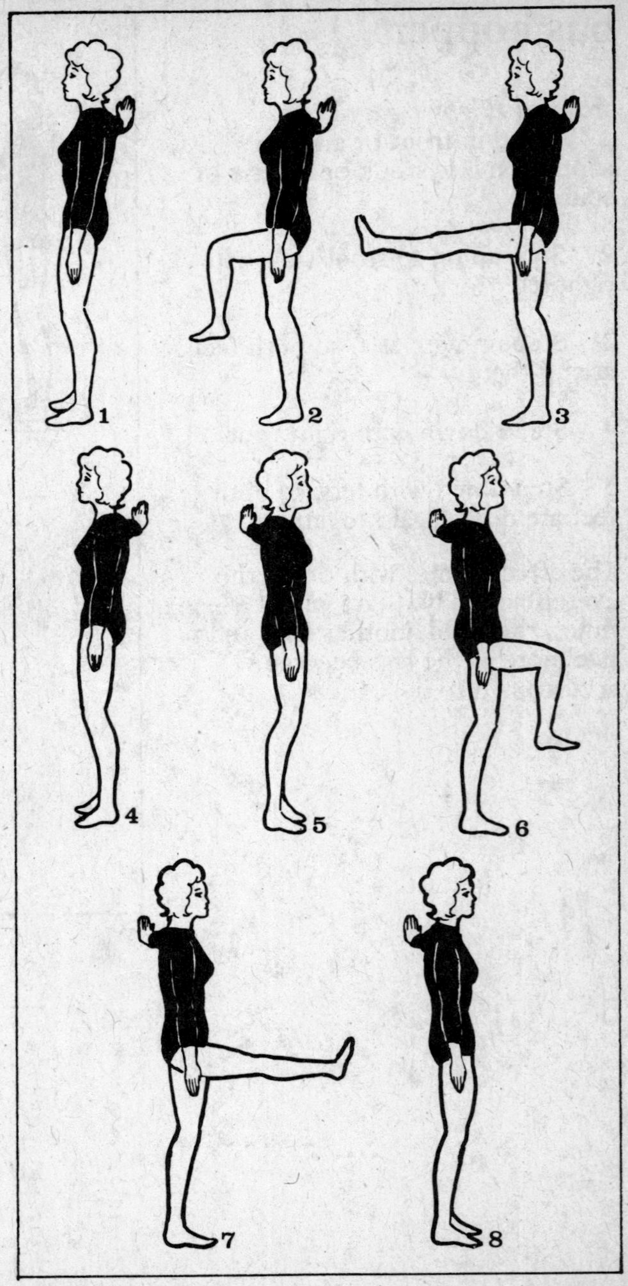

constabulary bends

front of thigh   harder

1 Stand with palms resting on thighs, feet apart.

2 Raise yourself up on your toes.

3 Bend knees and, pushing them outwards, lower to a sitting position.

4 Up on your toes again.

5 Return to the standing position.

Carry out the above sequence five times, slowly. Then do the following movements five times, slowly.

6 Raise yourself up on your toes.

7 Bend the knees, pushing them outwards. Lower the body till you are sitting on your heels.

8 Raise yourself up on your toes.

9 Lower the heels to the ground.

Gradually increase by one bend to each set of five, to a maximum of 10 sitting bends, plus 10 'to heel' bends.

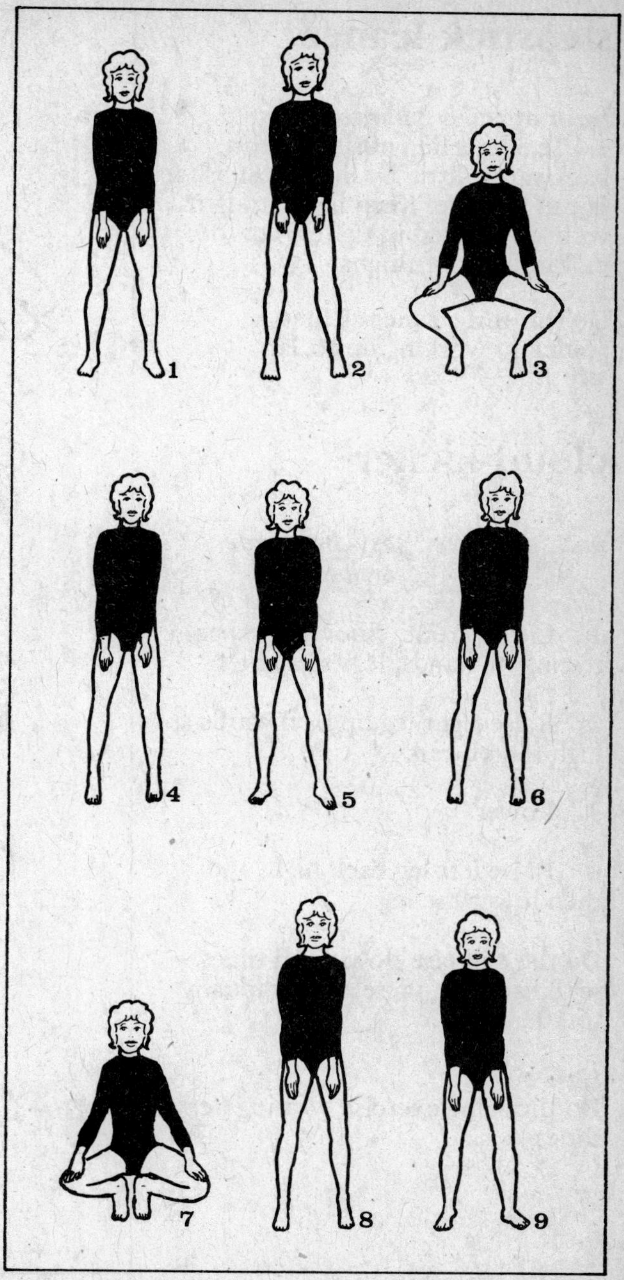

slapstick leaner

front of thigh   *harder*

1 In a kneeling position, lean backwards, little by little, just as far as can manage. Keep back straight, with seat pulled in tight. Feel the pull in front of thighs.

Do this three times as first, gradually working up to 10.

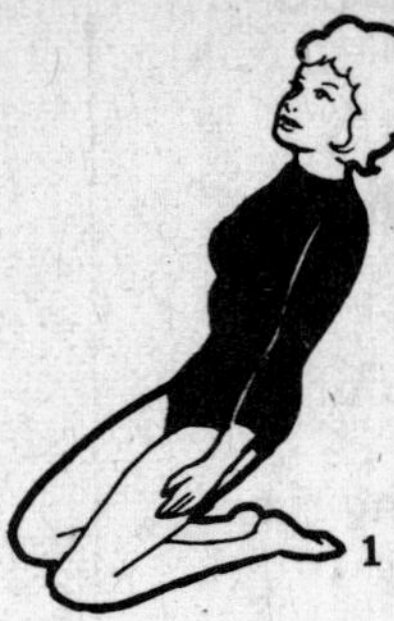

cloud kicker

back of thigh   *easy and harder versions*

Easy

1 Lie on front, elbows bent, chin resting on hands, legs straight.

2 Raise right leg up backwards as high as you can.

3 Lower.

4 Raise left leg back high, and then lower the leg.

Do the exercise slowly, 10 times with each leg, increasing gradually to 10.

Hard

Do the same exercise wearing heavy shoes.

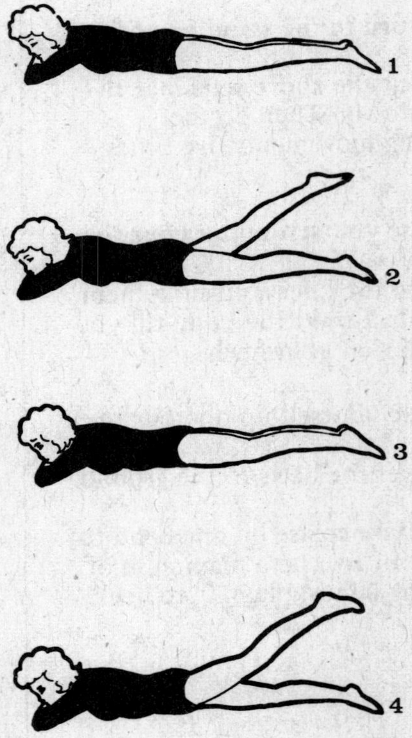

splits with a bounce

backs of thighs *harder*

1 Kneel.

2 Stretch right leg out straight.

3 Place a hand on the floor on either side of the body, for support. Stretch left leg back so that you are in a 'splits' position.

4 Using heel of right foot and toe of left foot as leverage, bounce left knee on floor 10 times.

Continued overleaf

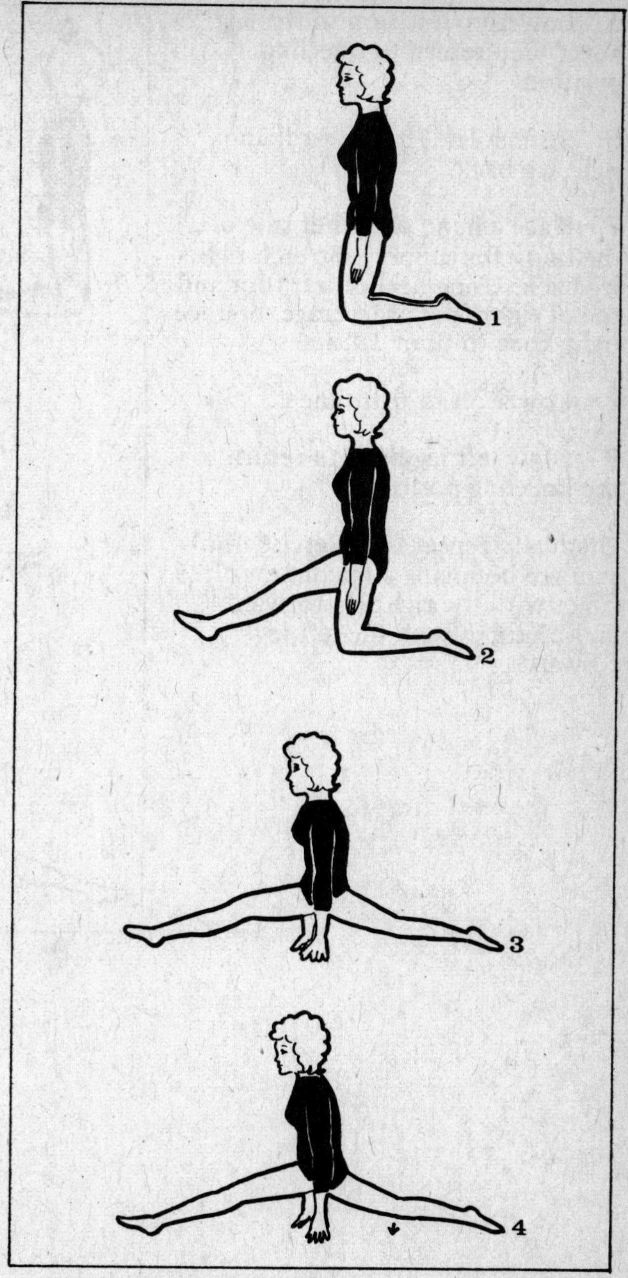

5 Lower yourself on to the left knee, then return to kneeling position.

6 Stretch left leg forward, and right leg back.

7 Place a hand on either side of the body for support. Stretch right leg back. Using heel of left foot and toe of right foot as leverage, bounce right knee to floor 10 times.

8 Lower on to right knee.

9 Draw left leg back to return to the kneeling position.

Gradually repeat the exercise until you are bouncing a maximum of 25 times with the right leg forward, and 25 times with the left leg forward.

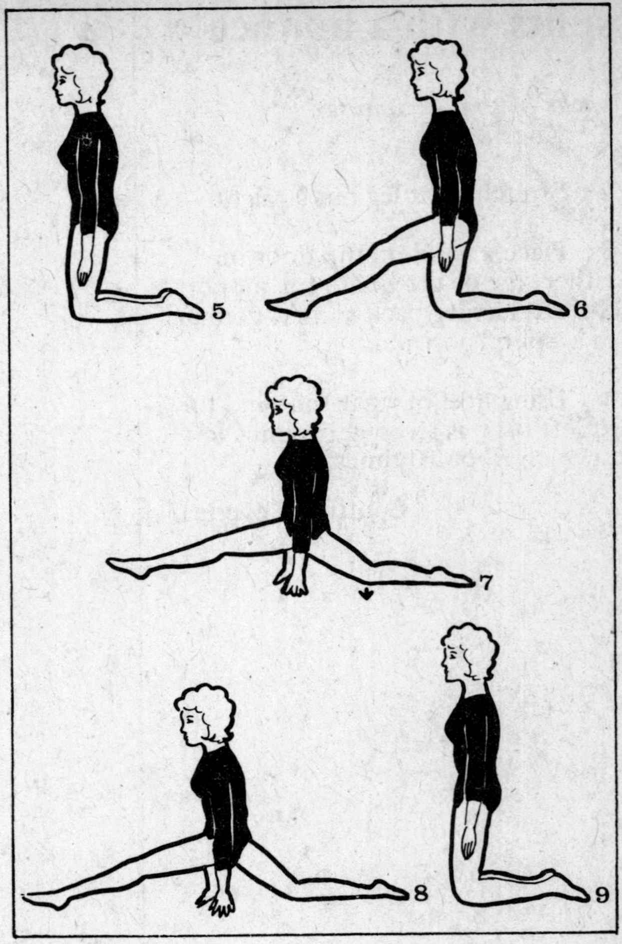

cushion clutch

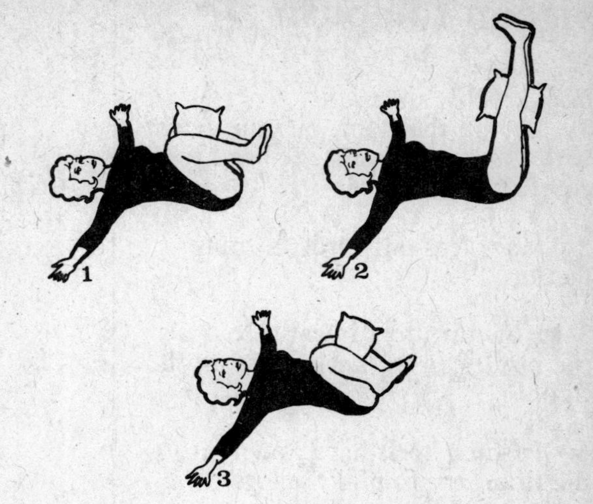

inner thighs *easier*
1 Lie on back, arms out to sides. With a cushion between knees, fold knees to stomach and squeeze cushion with knees.

2 Raise legs straight up, still gripping cushion with knees.

3 Do the knees-bend to the stomach again, then lower the legs.

Start by doing the exercise 10 times, increasing to 12 and then to 15. Progress to two sets of 10, with a rest in between.

nutcracker

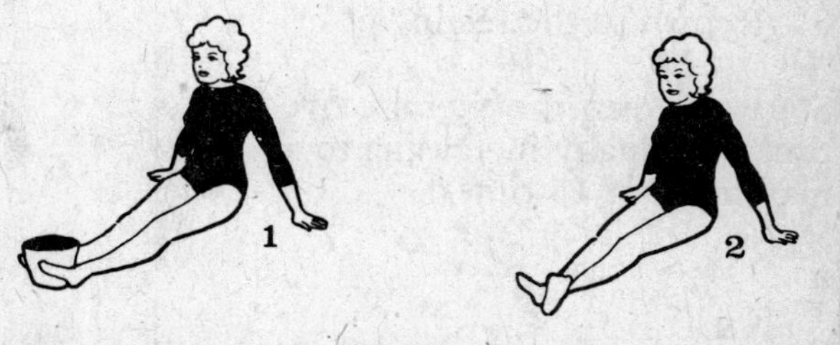

inner thighs *harder*
You need: a round basket, bin or cushion, about 10 to 16 inches in diameter.

1 Sit on floor, legs out straight, basket between feet, arms balancing at sides. Squeeze the legs together, trying to squash the basket. The pressure should be on the inner thighs.

2 Remove the basket, and cross the feet at the ankles. Try with your leg muscles to tug your legs apart while keeping the ankles firmly crossed. The feet will push against each other and you will feel the pull in the thigh muscles. Keep the back straight throughout.

Do the whole movement three times to begin with, gradually increasing by one to a maximum of 10.

pigeon toe push

inside thighs easy

1 Lay on the floor, on your back, with the hands under the head for comfort.

2 Move legs outwards, turning feet out.

3 Now turn feet inwards so that the insides of the heels press on the floor.

4 Pushing heels hard down into the floor, try to pull the legs together while resisting the movement. You will realise if you are pushing and pulling hard enough by the pull inside your thighs.

5 Return to the resting position.

Start by doing the exercise five times, gradually increasing to a maximum of 15 times.

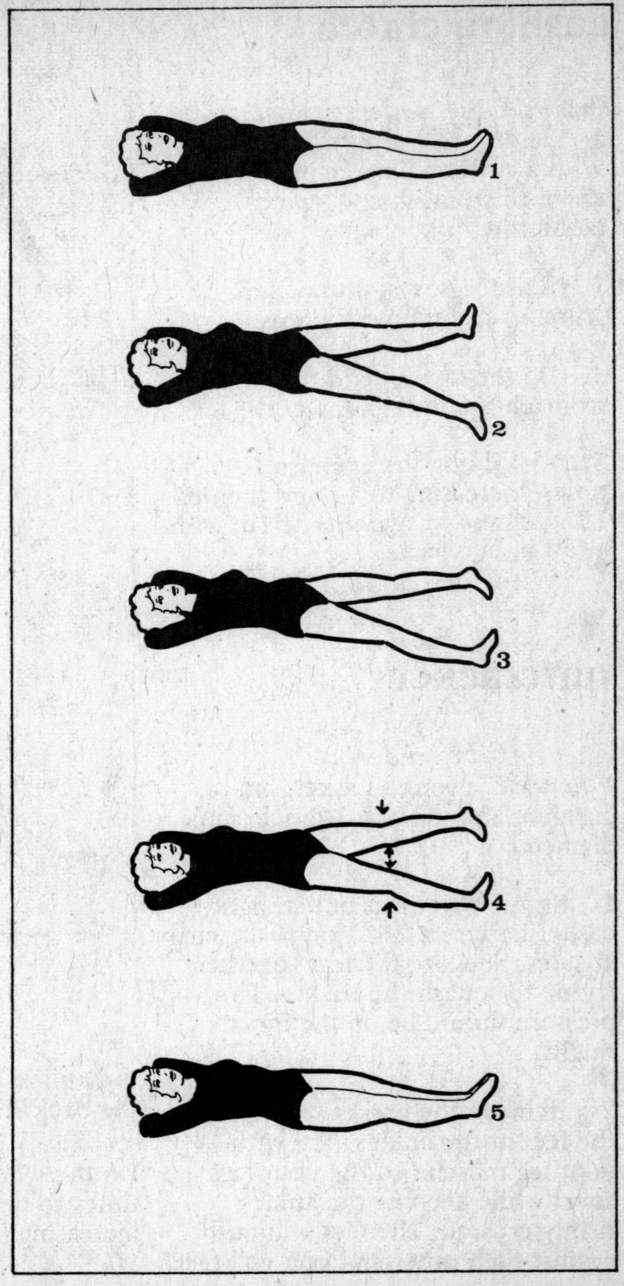

air ballet

inside thighs *harder*

1 Lay on back, with legs straight and arms out at shoulder level.

2 Bend knees on to stomach.

3 Straighten legs in the air.

4 Turn in toes, so that they touch.

5 Split legs wide to sides in the air, with the feet still turned in.

6 Turn the toes out and draw legs together.

7 Lower the legs and relax in the first position.

Do the exercise 10 times, working up to 15, then 20.

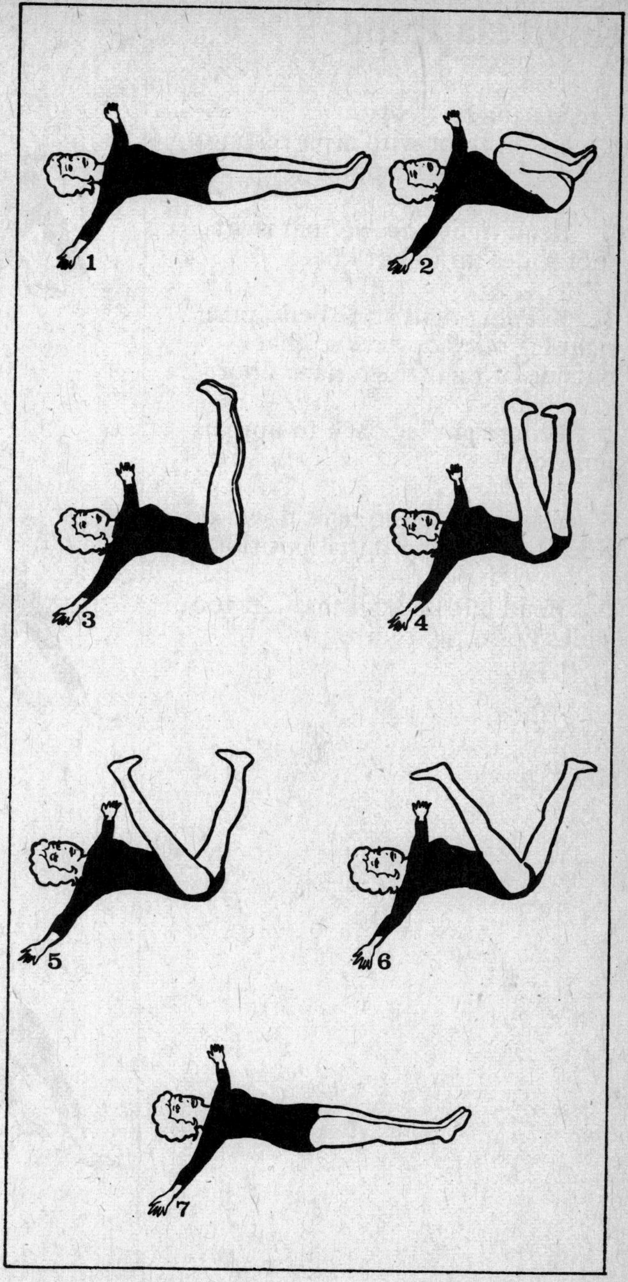

thigh slapping

outside thighs easy

1 Sit on floor with arms resting behind body for support.

2 Bend right knee so that right foot slides up to left knee.

3 Keeping right knee bent, push right leg out sideways so that outside of right thigh slaps floor.

4 Bring right leg back to upright position.

5 Slap right leg straight down on floor to return to initial position.

6 Bend left knee so that left foot slides up to right knee.

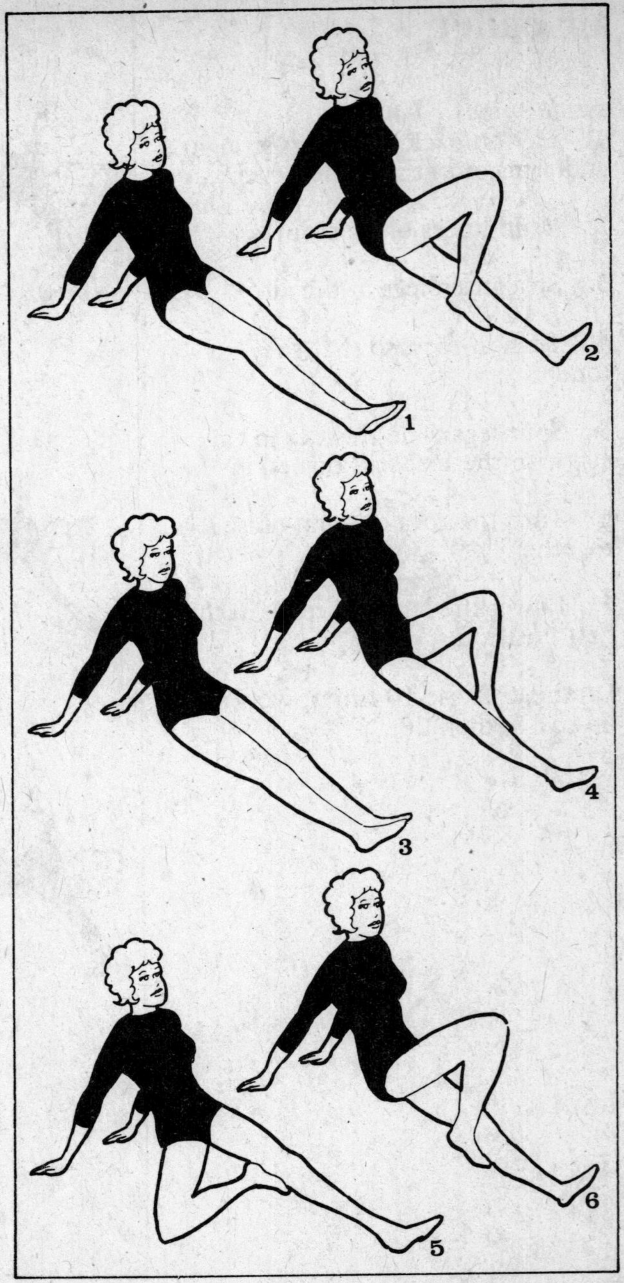

7 Keeping left knee bent, push left leg out sideways so that outside of left thigh slaps floor.

8 Bring left leg back to upright position.

9 Slap left leg straight down on floor to return to initial position.

Do the exercise 10 times, working up to 15, 20 and finally 30 times with each leg.

lean easy

outside thighs: easier for 'jodhpur' bulge

1 Stand sideways to a wall, resting right hand against wall for support. Bend knee of outside leg to the side. Raise until hips and legs are at a right angle, with the leg bent in front. Circle leg from the knee, anti-clockwise, keeping the thigh still.

2 Now take up a position with the left hand against the wall and the right leg raised. Repeat the exercise.

Do the exercise 10 times, increasing by two times gradually up to 20.

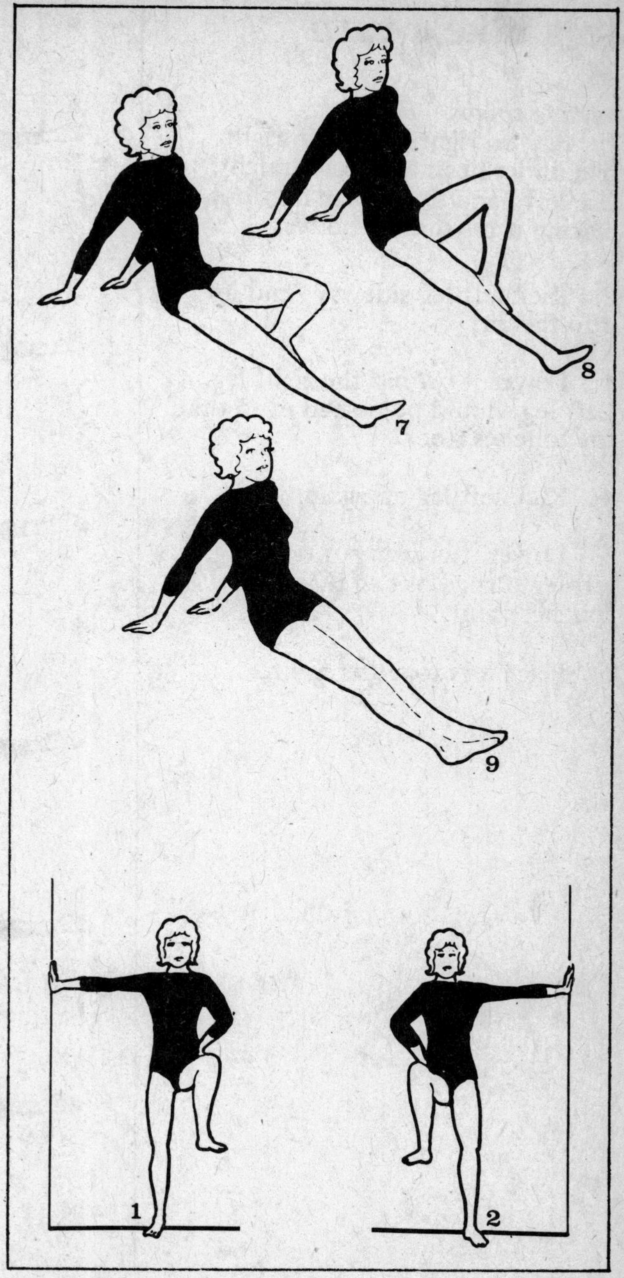

legs take a turn

outside thighs *hard*

1 Lay on right side, with right arm under head and legs straight. Use left hand to balance on floor, placing it in front of body.

2 Kick left leg sideways and up into the air.

3 Lower it *behind* the right leg. Left leg should be turned in so that toe touches floor.

4 Kick left leg up again.

5 Lower it in *front* of right leg, left leg turned out so that heel touches floor.

6 Place legs together again.

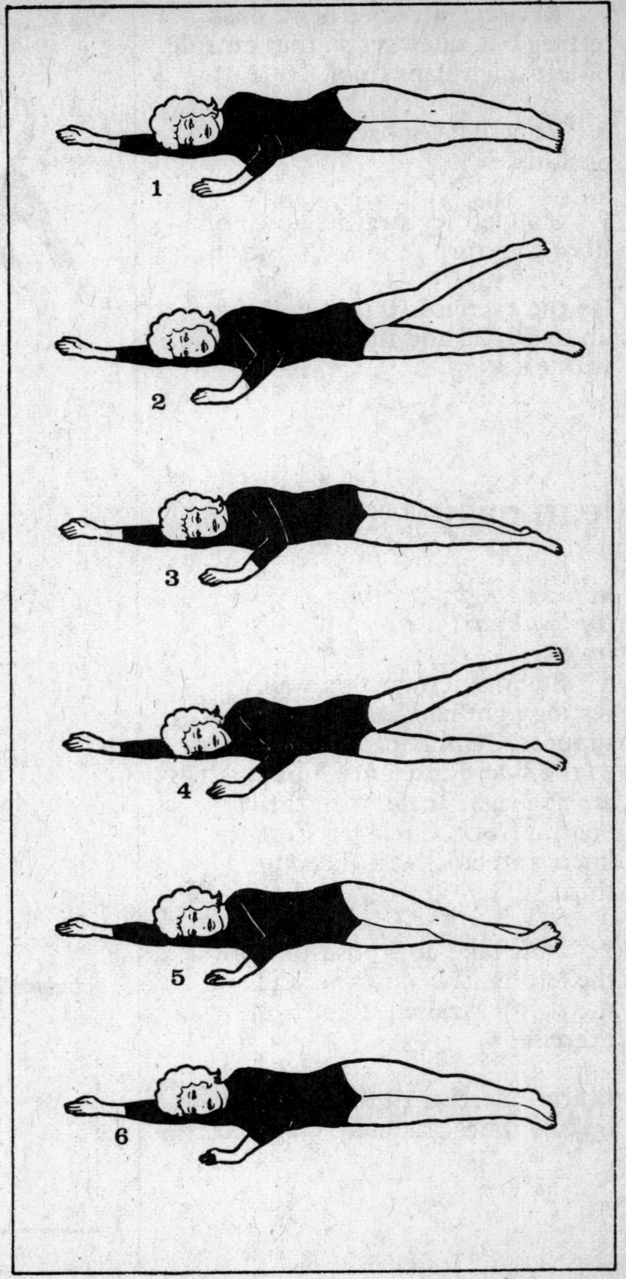

7 Raise right leg in air.

8 Lower right leg *behind* left, turning it inwards so that the toe touches the floor.

9 Raise right leg sideways into the air.

10 Lower right leg in *front* of left, with leg turned out so that the heel touches the floor.

11 Place legs together again.

Do the exercise fast 10 times, working up to 20 times for each leg.

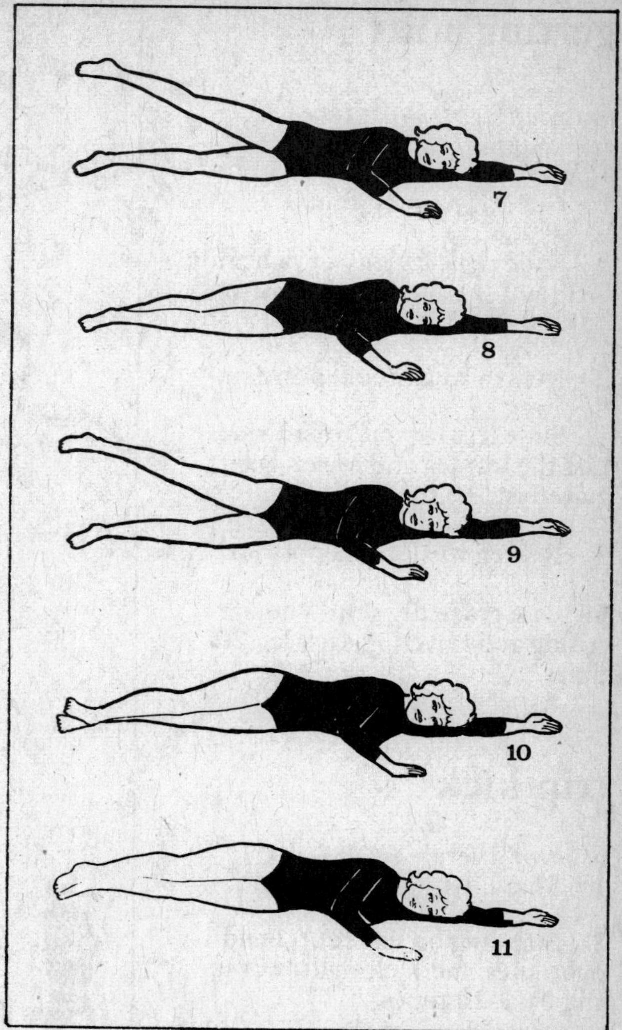

getting a lift

outside thighs: *harder*
for 'jodhpur'
bulge

1 Get down on all fours.

2 Slide right leg out to right side. Lift right leg and lower again quite fast, 10 times.

3 Return to all fours position.

4 Slide left leg out to left side. Lift the left leg and lower again quite fast, 10 times.

5 Return to all fours position.

Increase gradually until you are raising and lowering each leg 20 times.

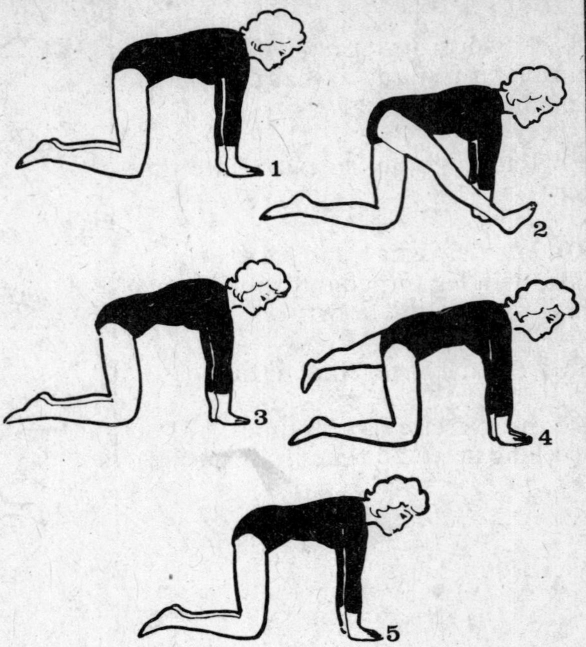

trip kick

front of knees *easy*

1 Stand, with feet together.

2 Standing on left foot, bend right knee and kick right foot up and back 20 times.

3 Put feet together.

4 Kick left foot up and back 20 times.

5 Put feet together again.

Do the exercise 20 times.

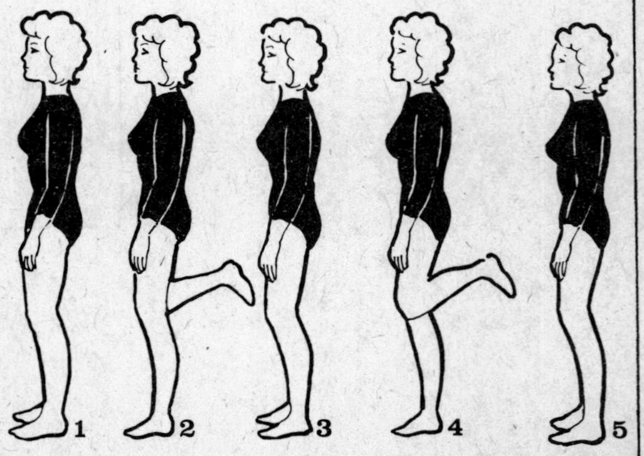

knee claps

knees easier

1 Sit straight on a hard chair. Hold on lightly, with hands on either side and feet slightly apart.

2 Clap knees together twice.

3 Straighten right knee so that the right leg is straight out in front with the heel only resting on the floor.

4 Raise right leg, keeping the knee straight.

5 Lower.

6 Straighten left knee, so that the leg is out in front, and the heel just touches the floor.

Continued overleaf

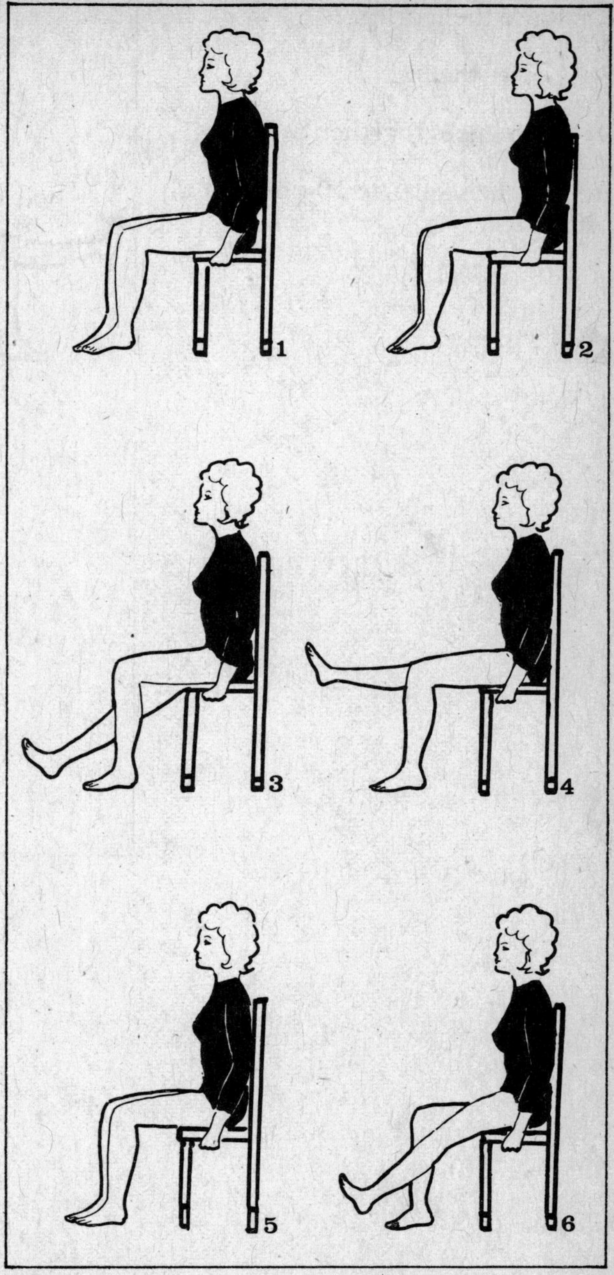

7 Raise the left leg.

8 Lower the leg.

9 Clap knees together twice.

Repeat the sequence 10 times, at a brisk pace.

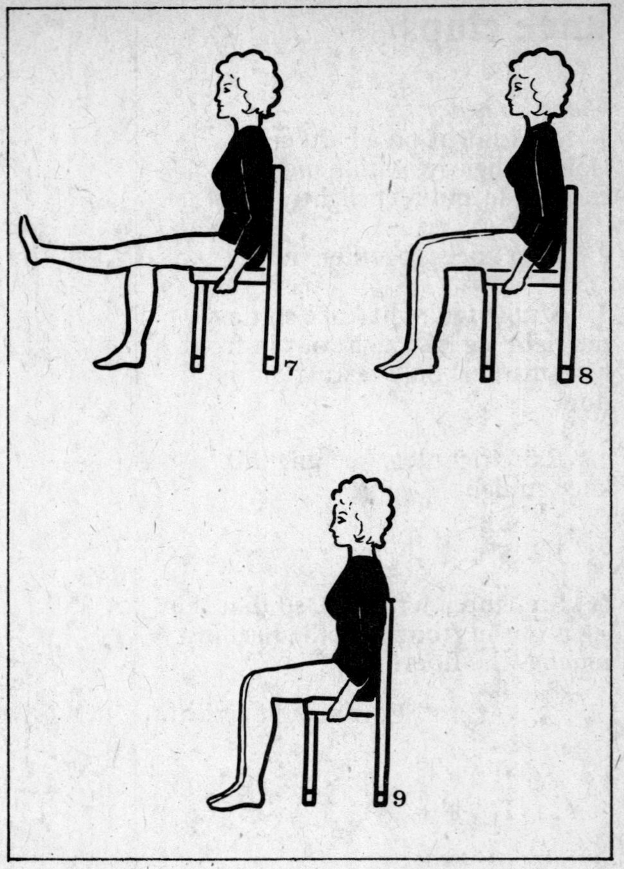

knee bounce

knees harder

1 Sit on floor, feet spread wide in a 'V'. Balance on hands, resting them behind you.

2 Bend knees slightly.

3 Stretch legs.

4 Bend knees.

5 Stretch legs.

6 Bend knees.

On the stretch, bounce the backs of the knees on the floor, and draw heels slightly in towards you on the bend.

7 Put legs together, straight out in front. Bounce backs of knees twice on the floor.

Do the exercise 10 times.

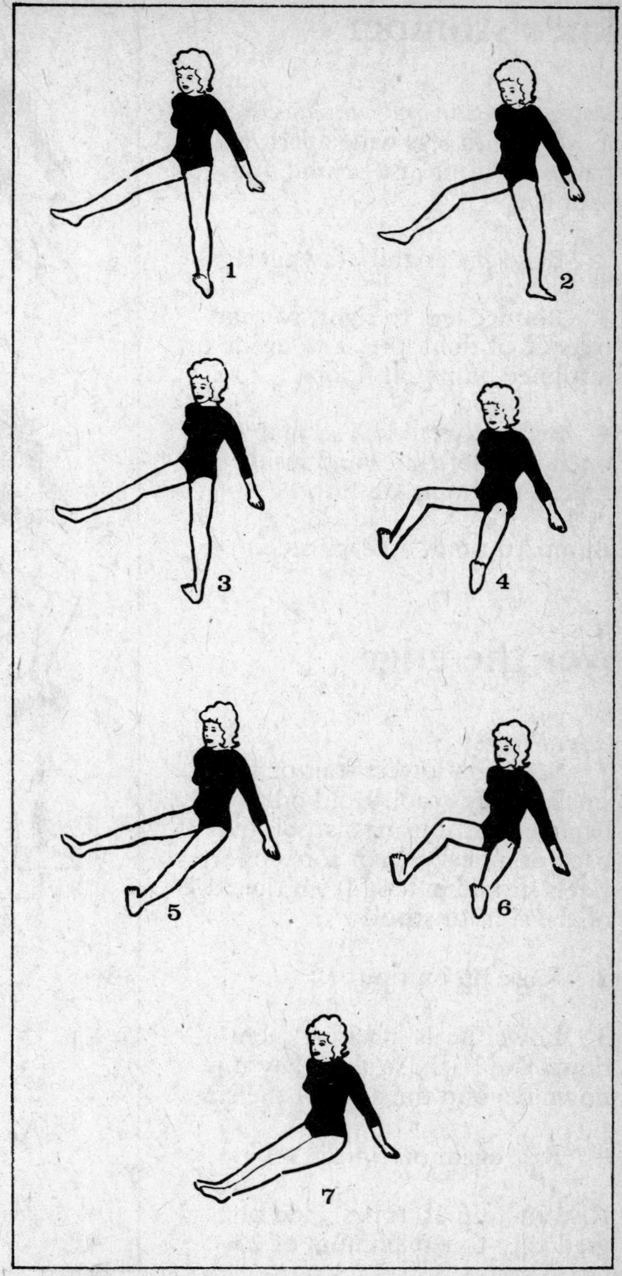

knee stomper

knees — inside and outsides *easy*
1 Sit, with legs wide apart, and hands on floor just behind you, for support.

2 Bend knees and draw up legs.

3 Bounce legs to right, so that outside of right knee and inside of left knee bump on floor.

4 Swing legs to left so that outside of left knee and inside of right knee bump on floor.

Bump 10 times on each side.

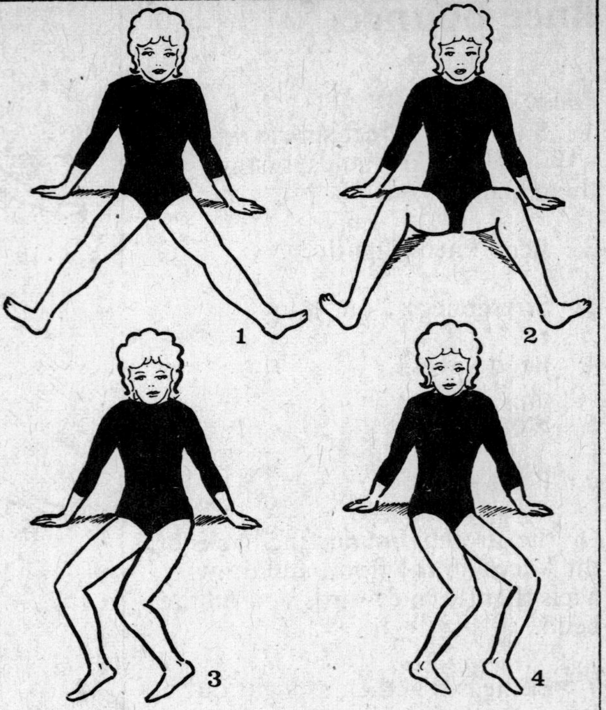

over the edge

calves *easy*
1 Stand on lowest stair or on a small sturdy stool. Hold on to banister, or, if using a stool, the back of a heavy chair for support. Heels should extend from the edge of the stair or stool.

2 Raise up on tip-toe.

3 Lower heels, pushing them down and back, so that they dip down beyond the edge of the stair.

4 Rise again on tip-toe.

Rise and dip 10 times. Add one gradually to a maximum of 25.

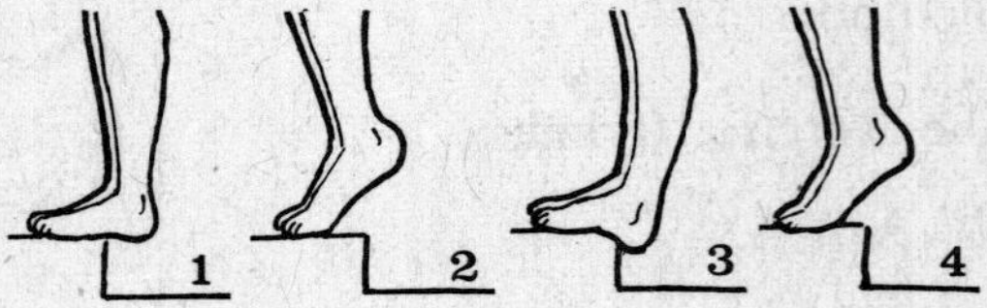

ins and outs

calves easier

1 Stand, holding the back of chair for support.

2 Turn feet inwards.

3 Rise on the toes.

4 Lower heels, feet still inwards.

5 Swivelling from knees, turn toes out.

6 Rise on toes.

7 Lower heels.

8 Swivel feet in to repeat the exercise.

Do the whole exercise fast, 10 times. Push from the feet, keeping the seat under.

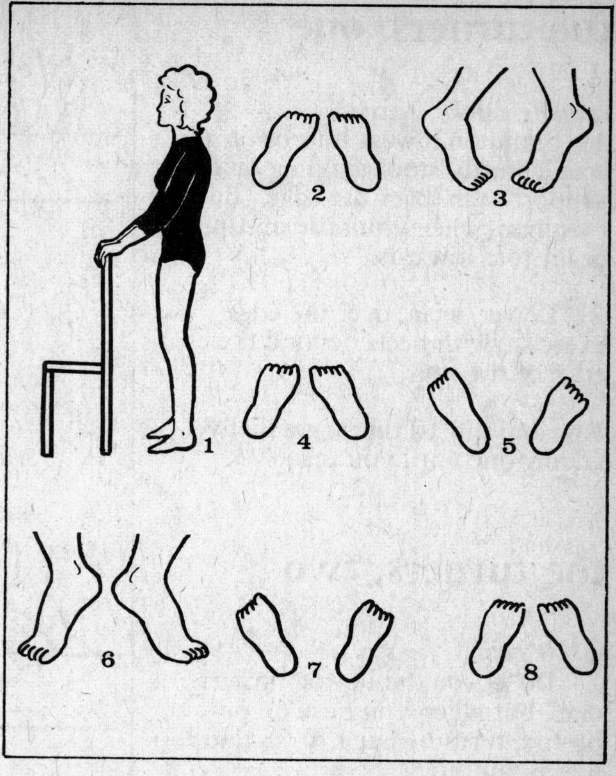

toe turners, one

outside calves   easy

1 Stand on lowest stair or on a small, sturdy stool, holding on for support as in 'over the edge'. But this time, when you raise on tip-toe, point toes inwards.

2 Lower, as in 'over the edge' exercise, with heels beyond the edge of the stair.

Rise and dip 10 times, gradually adding one until you reach 25.

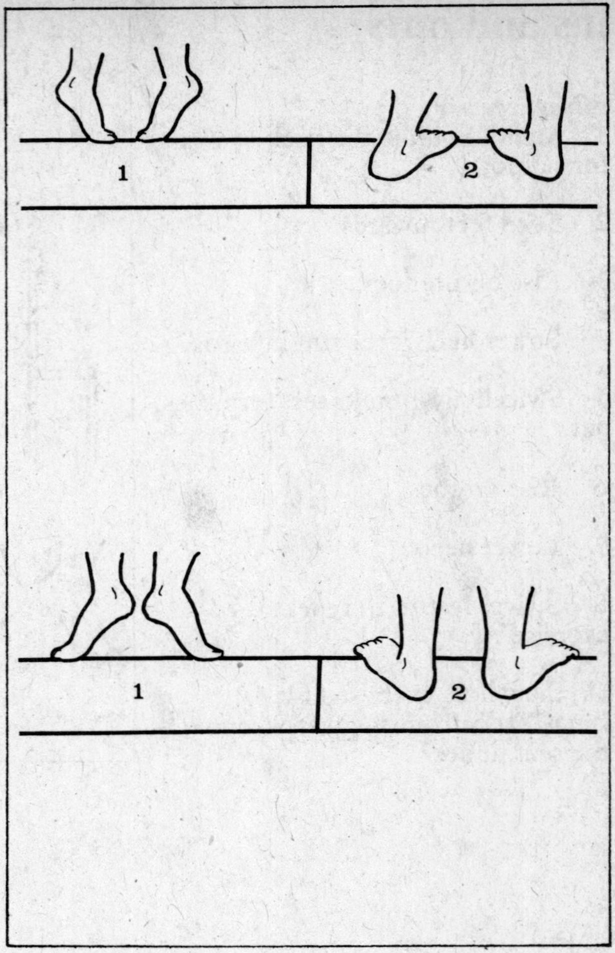

toe turners, two

inside calves   easy

1 Do as you did in 'toe turners one', but when you raise up on tip-toe, turn the heels *in*, so that toes point out.

2 Lower. You need to stand with feet about a foot apart, in order to be able to turn heels inwards comfortably.

ups and downs

calves *harder*

1 Stand, holding back of chair, with feet 18 inches apart. Turn feet slightly outwards, and keep back straight.

2 Rise on the balls of the feet.

3 Squat, still on the toes, and still keeping the back straight. Keep seat well tucked in. Knees will automatically lower over toes.

4 Rise on toes.

5 Lower heels.

Do the exercise six times. Later, increase to eight, and then to 10.

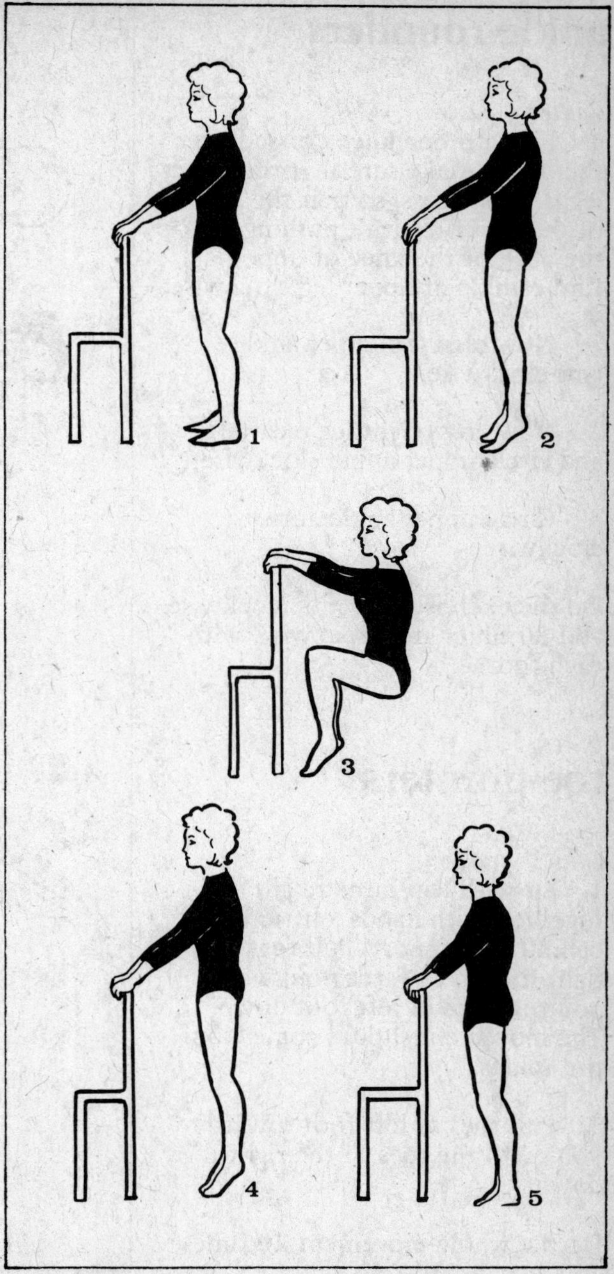

ankle rounders

ankles *easy*
1 Sit with one knee crossed over the other. Make sure that the upper leg is well across, so that the knee of the lower leg isn't pushing into the back of the knee of upper leg. Circle ankle of upper leg clockwise.

2 Now turn the upper ankle anti-clockwise.

3 Now cross right leg over left and circle upper ankle clockwise.

4 Circle upper ankle anti-clockwise.

Do the exercise 20 times clockwise and 20 times anti-clockwise, with each foot.

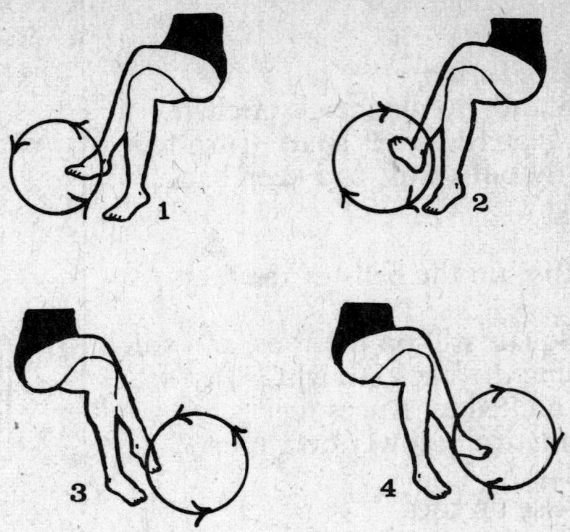

toe pointers

ankles *easy*
1 Sit with legs out straight and together, with hands a little way behind for support. Pull toes of right foot in towards you, while pointing toes of left foot down. The movement should come from the ankles.

2 Pull toes of left foot towards you, with the toes of the right foot down.

Do the whole movement 20 times.

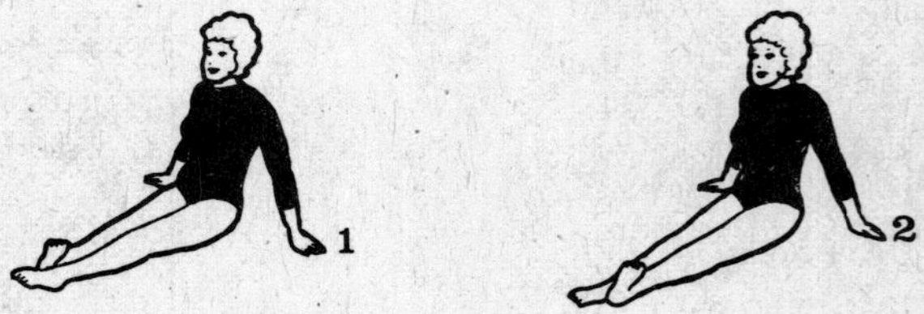

foot flips

ankles harder

1 Sit down on floor, with legs out straight, feet about a foot apart and hands behind for support.

2 Roll the feet to the right so that the *outside* of the right foot and the *inside* of the left foot touch the floor together.

3 Roll feet to the left so that the *outside* of the left foot and the *inside* of the right foot touch the floor. The impetus should come from the ankles.

Repeat five times, working up to 10.

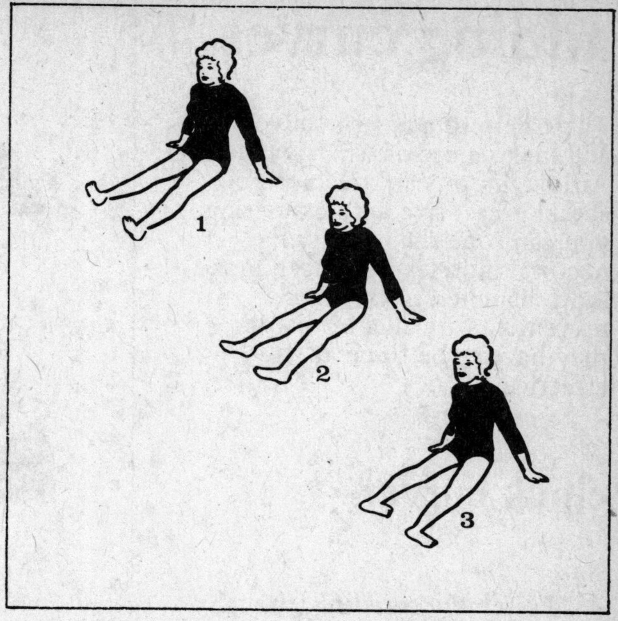

adding curves

These help to add womanly curves and make more of what you've got. Although you can't change your actual breast size with exercising, you can tone the underlying pectoral muscles which can make it look shapelier. Sorry, these movements are all a bit harder – they have to be to be at all effective.

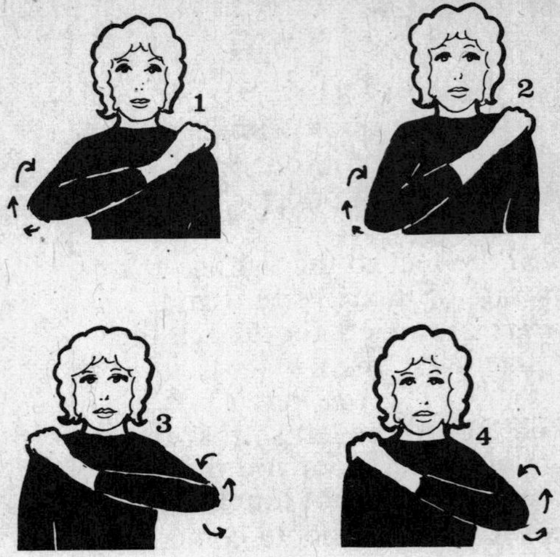

clock curver

bust

1 Preferably standing (though you can sit), place right hand on left shoulder. Keep elbow well up. Draw five clockwise circles with the elbow.

2 Now do five anti-clockwise circles with the elbow.

3 Place left hand on right shoulder, with elbow well up, and draw five clockwise circles with left elbow.

4 Then five anti-clockwise circles with the left elbow.

piston pusher

bust
You need: A weight to hold in each hand – a household tool or a can of vegetables will do – of about 3 lbs. It should be comfortable enough to swing around without dropping.

1 Standing erect, with feet apart, hold weights straight out in front.

2 Pull weights back behind you, elbows down, breathing in.

3 Push weights out in front, breathing out.

The exercise is a fast one, and should be done briskly. Five times at first, building to 20.

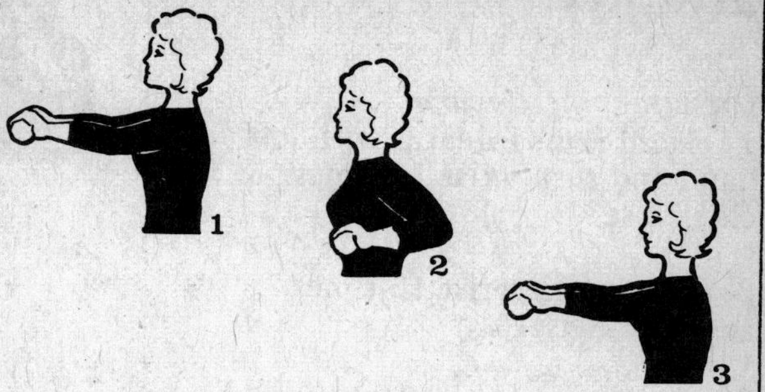

me, Tarzan

arms (and good for salt cellars)
1 Stand with feet wide apart. Raise arms to shoulder level, with palms facing front.

2 Holding this hand position, clench fists.

3 Resist, as if someone is pulling you back, and draw fists in to touch shoulders. Imagine you are squeezing the sides of the bust together. Bounce fists twice at the shoulders before extending the arms slowly against the imagined resistance.

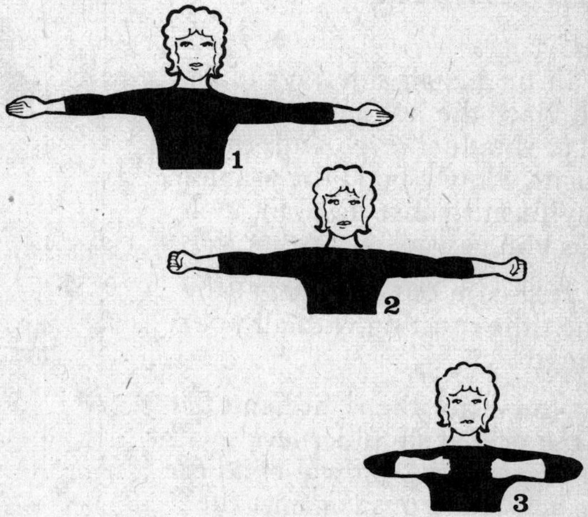

On extension, really tighten the elbows and brace the shoulders, with the arms really pulling back.

Do the exercise six to eight times.

arm jive

strengthening forearm

1 Hold right forearm with left hand and turn wrist 10 times clockwise.

2 Turn right wrist 10 times anti-clockwise.

3 Reverse arms, and turn left wrist 10 times clockwise.

4 Turn left wrist 10 times anti-clockwise.

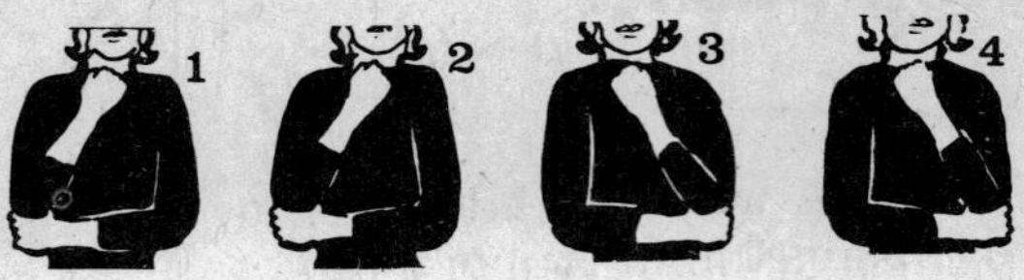

wall resister

arms

1 Sit on a chair sideways to a wall. Place the left hand flat on the wall at shoulder level, with the arm straight. Slowly bend the arm and really push against the wall, in as far as you can go.

2 Push arm out straight, at the same time resisting with all your strength.

3 Now place the right hand flat on the wall at shoulder level, with the arm straight. Slowly bend the arm and really push against the wall, resisting all the time.

4 Push the arm out straight, at the same time resisting as hard as you can.

Do the exercise five times. Later, do two sets of five, then three and four sets of five.

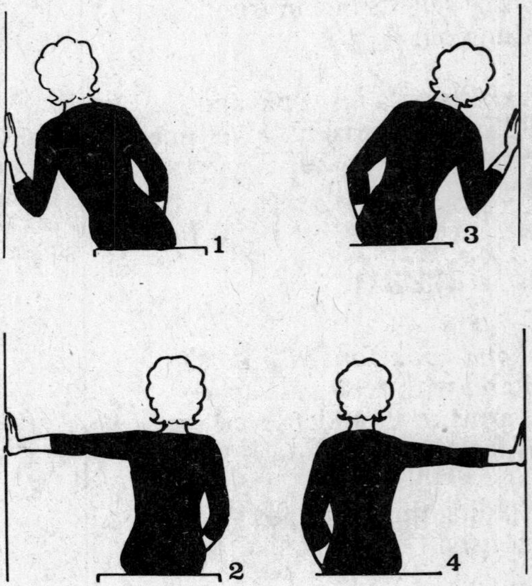

toe tapper

calves

1 Stand sideways to a wall, supporting yourself with your right hand.

2 Point the left toe downwards, really bracing the leg and foot. Stretch the leg forward and hit the toe sharply on the floor twice.

3 Stretch the left leg backwards and bounce the toe twice on the floor behind.

4 Now turn around so that your left hand is supporting you against the wall.

5 Point the toe of the right foot downwards, bracing the foot. Stretch forward and hit the toe sharply on the floor, twice.

6 Stretch the right leg back, and bounce the toe twice on the floor behind.

Do the exercise slowly, keeping the legs and feet braced. Do it 10 times for each leg.

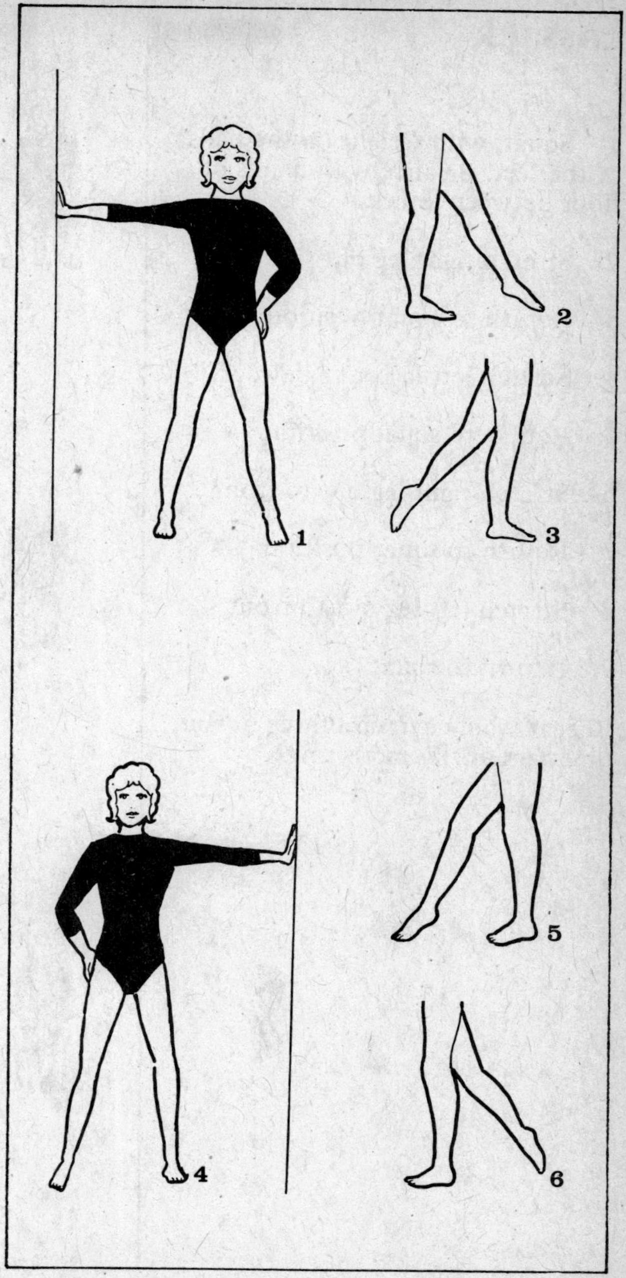

cossack

calves

1 Squat, with weight on the balls of the feet. Balance with hands on floor between knees.

2 Stretch right leg out sideways.

3 Return to squat position.

4 Stretch left leg out sideways.

5 Return to squat position.

6 Stretch right leg out to front.

7 Return to squat position.

8 Stretch left leg out to front.

9 Return to squat.

Repeat whole exercise three or four times, gradually increasing.

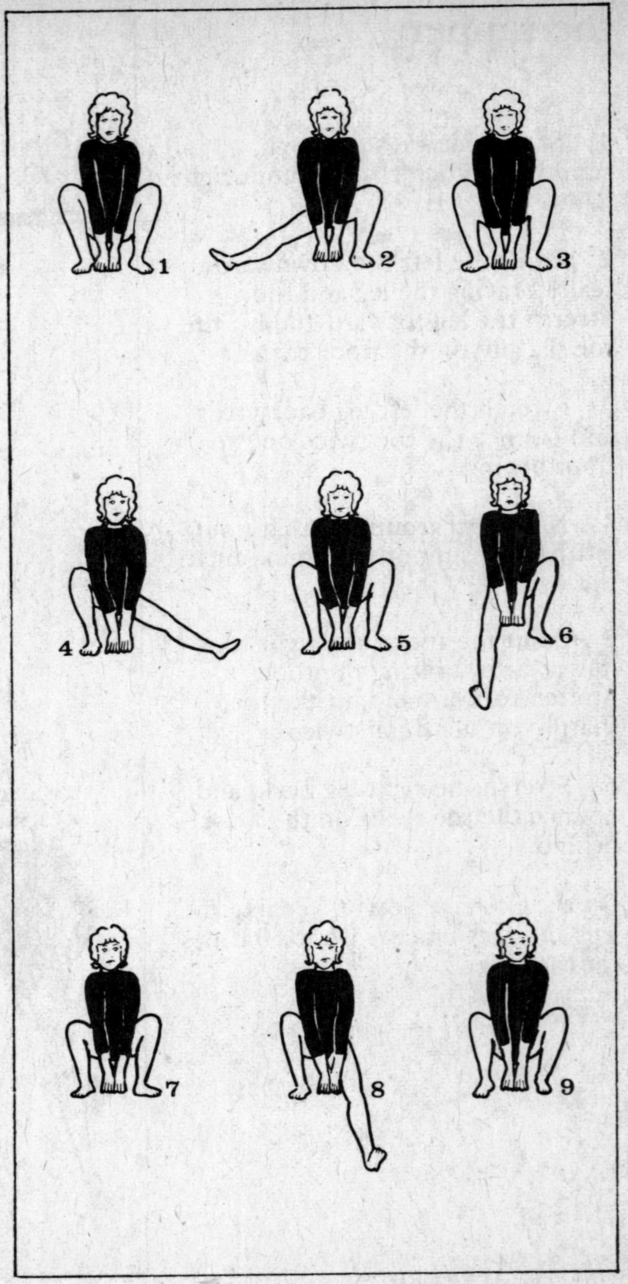

phantom fencer

all over legs

1 Stand with feet apart.

2 Raise arms to shoulder level.

3 Turning slightly to right, bend left knee and slide right foot towards the right. Sink as low as you can. Keep back straight, seat in. The left foot stays facing front. Bracing the legs, hold the position for a slow count of three gentle bounces.

4 Returning to starting position.

5 Turning slightly to the left, bend right knee, and slide left foot leftwards. Sink low, keeping back straight, and seat in. The right foot faces front. Hold for slow count of three.

6 Return to starting position.

Increase counts of three, and gradually 'sink' lower.

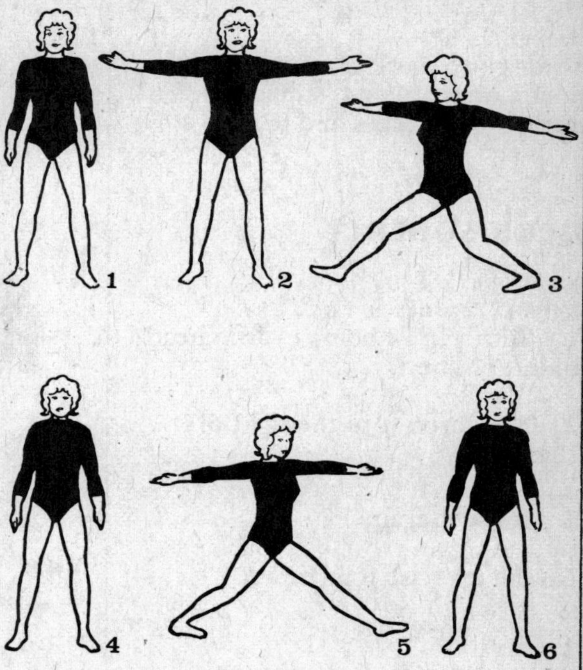

pushover

all over legs

1 Sitting at well supported table or desk – or another chair – place the feet inside the desk legs, and push as if trying to force the static legs apart. Hold for a count of three.

Do this three times to begin with, increasing gradually to 10.

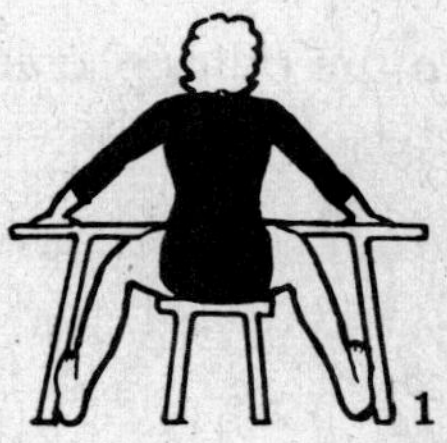

relaxers

These go to work on pressure points where mental strain converts into physical aches and pains.

neck soother

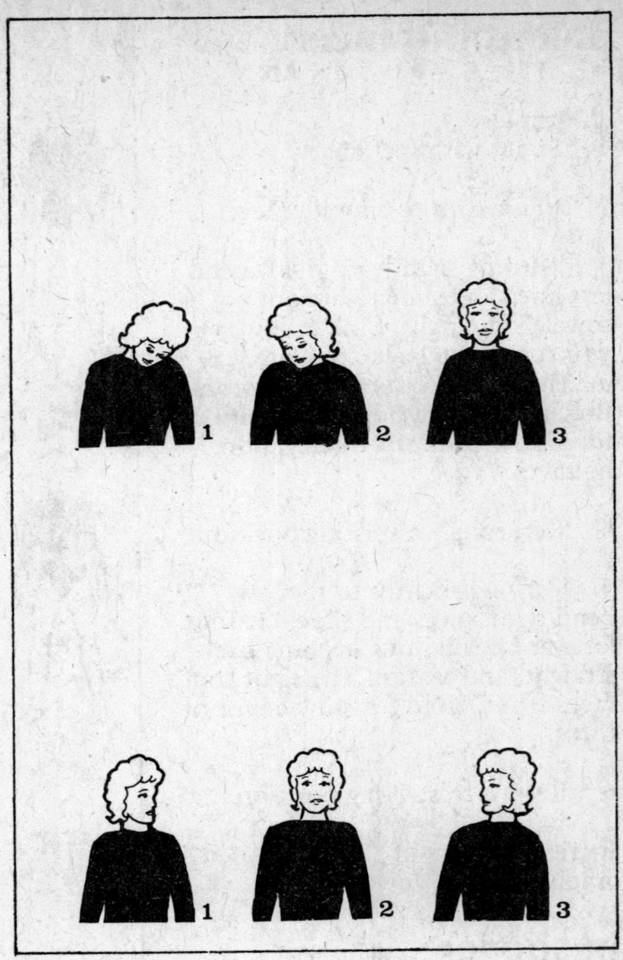

relieves tension in back of neck
1 With a *little* bounce, drop head to left of chest.

2 Now drop it to the right of chest.

3 Raise it again.

Do the exercise four times.

Wimbledon whirl

for a stiff neck
1 Imagine you are watching a game of tennis. Turn head to left hand player.

2 Turn front to the ball.

3 Turn right to the other player. And so on.

Do the exercise four to six times.

shrug off

for stiff shoulders

1 Simply shrug one shoulder at a time. But make it a really hard, shirty shrug. Do four to six shrugs with each shoulder.

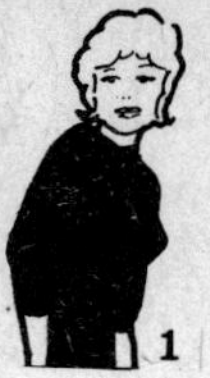

kingcup

relaxer for stiff jawline and teeth grinders

1 Rest elbows on firm surface, chin on hands. Push chin down on to heels of hands, while pushing heels of hands hard up to chin. Hold push for a slow count of six or eight. Do this twice.

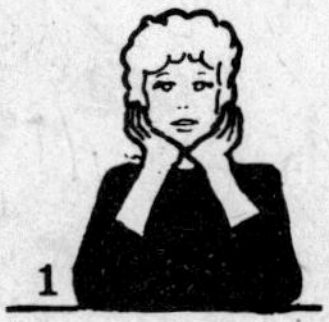

shimmy cat

to relax taut spine

1 Get on all fours, circle hips and waist. Get the feel by lifting up.

2 Go to right side and down.

3 Then to the left side and down.

Do six shimmies.

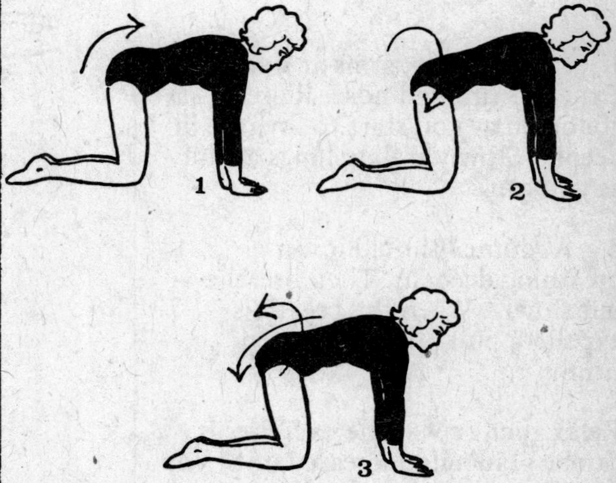

seagull

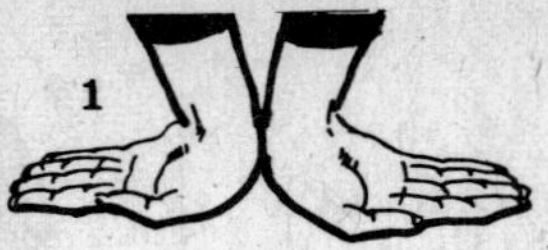

a flyer for stiff, achey wrists

1 Put wrists together. Flap hands like a bird's wings for between 30 seconds and a minute.

mock shampoo

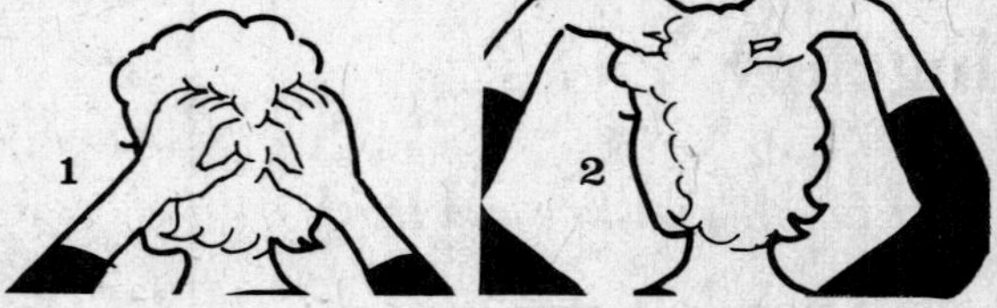

to relax scalp tight with tension

1 With thumbs at the nape of neck, spreadeagle hands and move (don't rub) flesh of scalp in little circular movements.

2 Work sideways and up towards forehead until all head is covered.

like-yoga breather

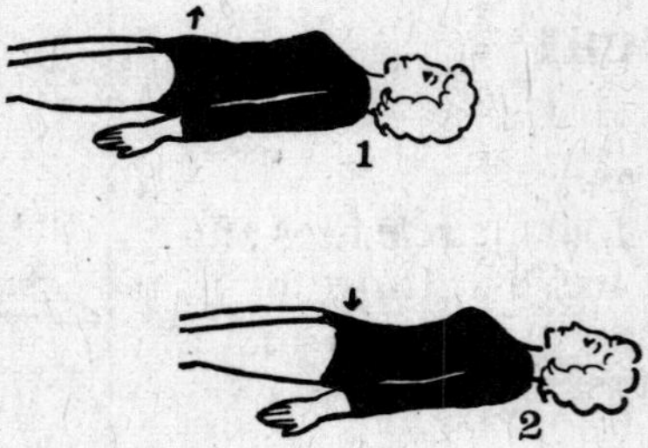

1 Lay on floor, arms at sides. Expel air through nose. Raise abdomen as you start to breathe in deeply. Slowly inflate lungs as fully as you can.

2 Abdomen should lower as breathing deepens. Then breathe out slowly. When the breath is expelled, pull in the abdomen firmly.

Relax then repeat the exercise. It can be gradually increased until you are doing it six or seven times.

jiffy liveners

These run the gamut from something for dedicated non-exercisers to quick perks for the jaded and fading.

first thing liveners for loafers

The five movements comprise a lazy-wake routine. If you are specially short on time or wind, do just the first and second exercise. The first should always be followed by the second to align muscles properly.

1 super stretch

1 Do the exercise as slowly as you like. Push away pillow. Stretch arms up. You are trying to touch the bedhead or wall, but it's just out of reach. At the same time point the toes so that there is one long stretch from fingers to toes.

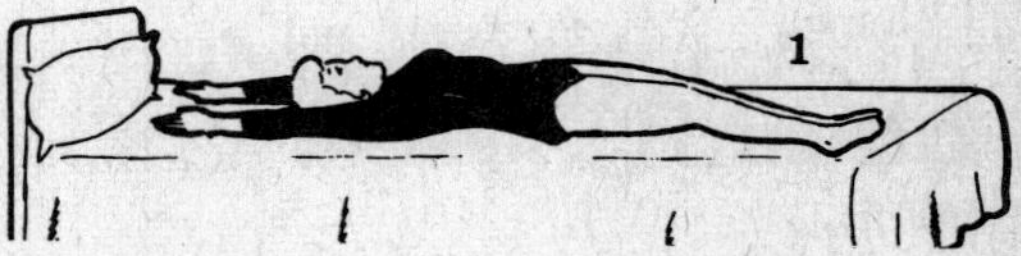
1

2 glad hug

1 Fold knees on to stomach – there's no hurry. Wrap arms around the knees and draw them into the abdomen, pulling in the abdomen at the same time. Once is enough.

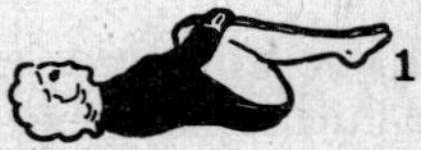
1

3 toe teaser

1 Get into a lying position.

2 and 3 Sit up and swing arms over to touch toes.

To make it easier, you can keep feet apart. Do the exercise four to six times.

4 a little grip

1 Swing legs over side of bed. Swing arms to grip edge of bed lightly on the right hand side.

2 Swing arms to grip the edge of the bed on the left hand side.

Repeat the exercise six to eight times.

5 cat curl

1 Sit on the edge of the bed, with the legs straight.

2 Begin with the hands on the thighs and slide them down to the toes, then up and off to the sides again.

The exercise should be slow and rhythmic. You are curling and uncurling and the hand sliding helps to control this.

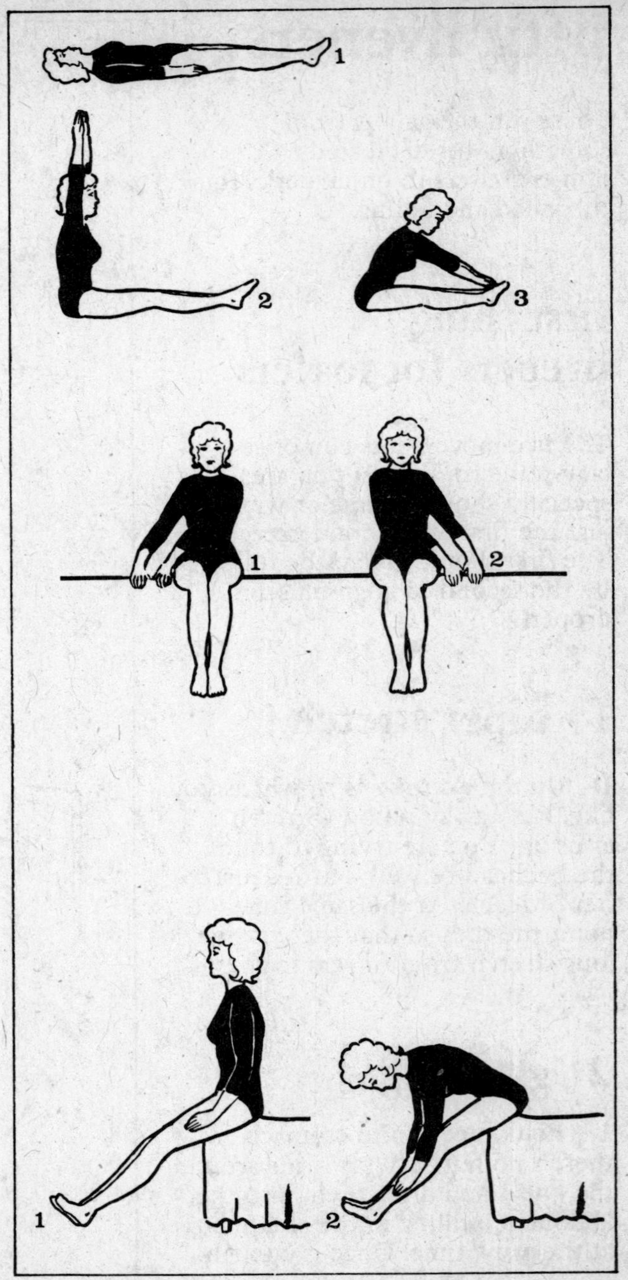

revivers for waking hours

rainbow chaser

stiff arms *easier*

1 With feet slightly apart, relax arms at sides.

2 Swing arms across body to the right.

3 Then put arms over the head . . .

4 . . . and down to the left.

Swing six circles to the left, and then six to the right.

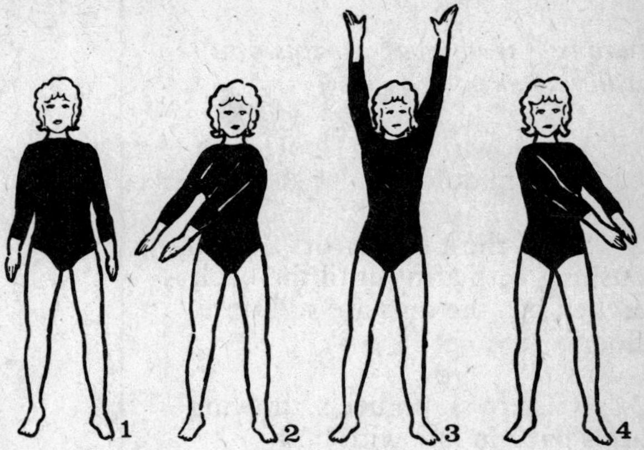

jumping bean

easier

You need: A bean bag or old sock filled with a pound or less of split peas, acorns, conkers, porridge oats, etc. Remember to put into a plastic bag before putting into sock.

1 Stand, and grip bag between feet. Maintaining grip, jump up and down 10 times.

2 Throw bag in air with one hand and catch with opposite hands. Do this 10 times.

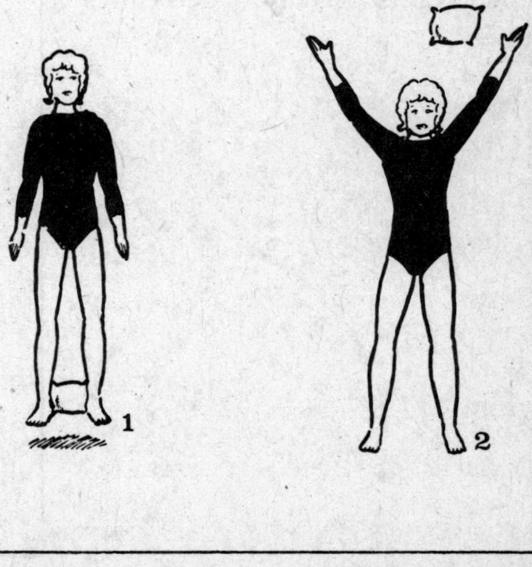

swan swoop

harder – if you can do this you're really awake

1 Lay down, facing floor, with hands palm down under shoulders.

2 Raise chest slowly off floor by pushing with arms until the back is arched but the hips are still on floor.

3 Raise to sit on heels, drawing arms back in line with body.

4 Rest forehead on floor, arms stretched forward, palms down.

5 Taking weight on hands, slide chin along just above floor . . .

6 . . . and body through and ahead of arms to lie flat on floor.

Do the exercise slowly, three times.

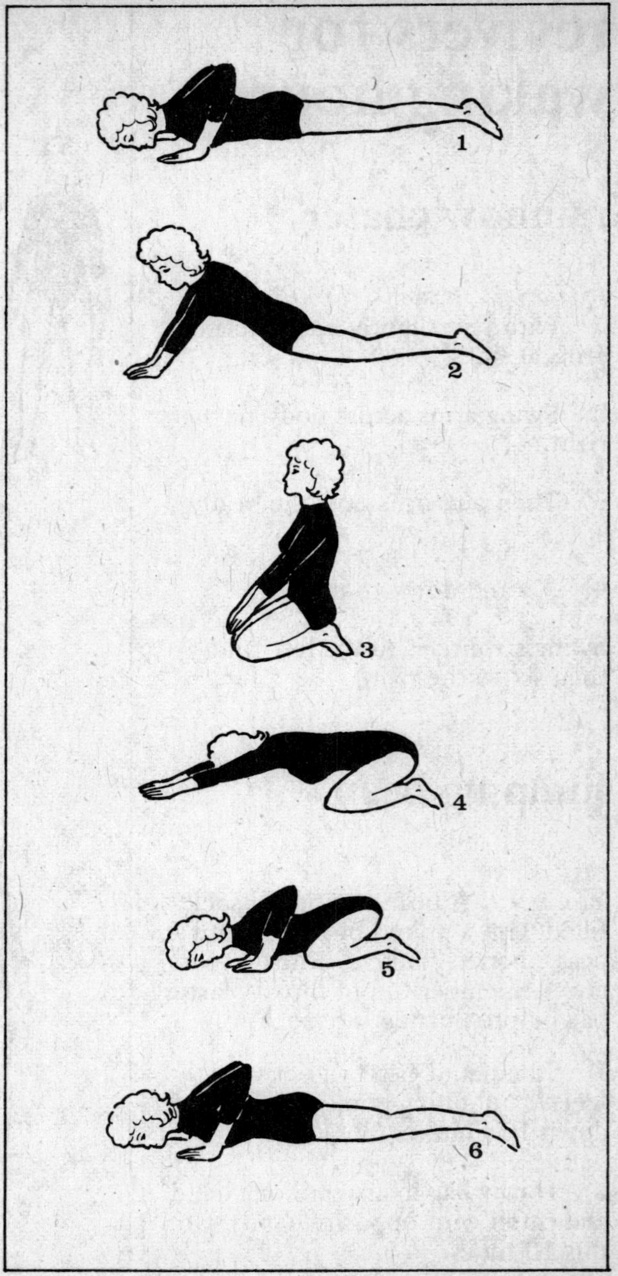

look younger – longer

Use these carefully modulated movements which help alleviate the physical give-aways.

walk tall

general stance

1 Stand against a straight wall. Try to line up spine with wall, touching with head, shoulder blades and seat. Take feet a little bit away, to help. Pull in chin: pull up from crown, as if a string were pulling you up.

2 Press against wall at all touching points, then push small of back against wall and relax.

Do exercise five to 10 times to get the feel of it. Try to maintain this posture when walking.

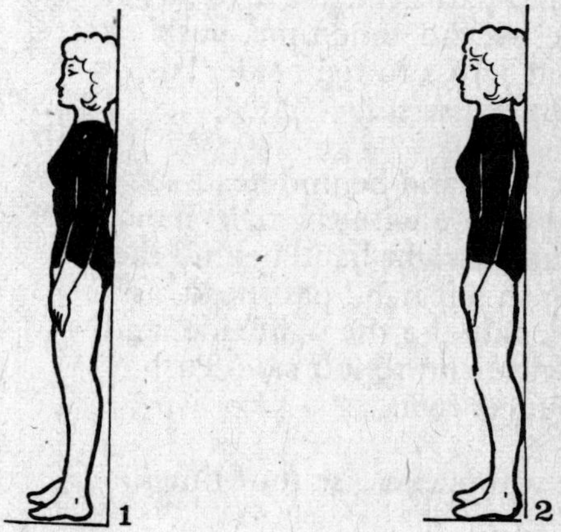

a little lift

sliding bosom

1 Sit at a table, arms straight, palms face down. Push down hard, keeping arms straight. Try to push table through floor. Hold for a count of 10.

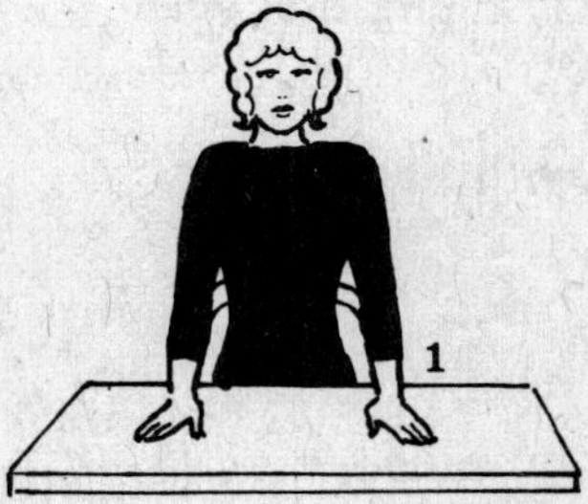

village pump

fat round upper back and shoulders (dowager's hump)

1 You can sit down for this. Put right hand behind head, resting head on palm, and put left hand behind back, with the back of hand touching middle of back. Hold the elbow back and keep bent. Push right hand past head as far to left as possible. At the same time, push left hand across to right side. Push, in a bounce, twice.

2 Put left hand behind head, as you did before with the right hand. Now put the right hand behind the back. Push left hand past head, as far as possible to the right side, and push right hand to left side. Push, in a bounce, twice.

Do the whole exercise four times.

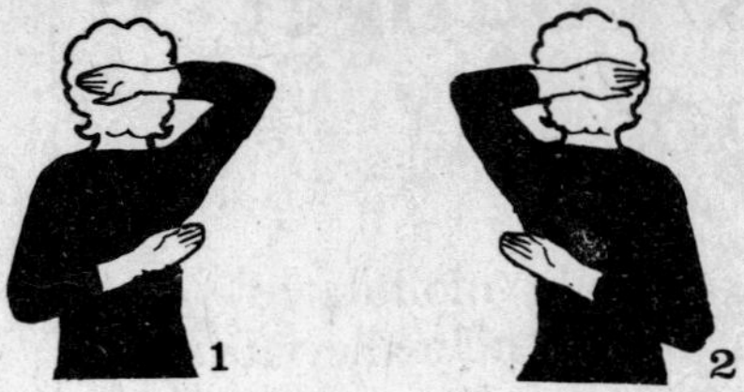

piano player

finger suppler

1 Sitting on a chair, use the thighs as a piano. Play them, first with fingers straight . . .

2 . . . then with fingers bent.

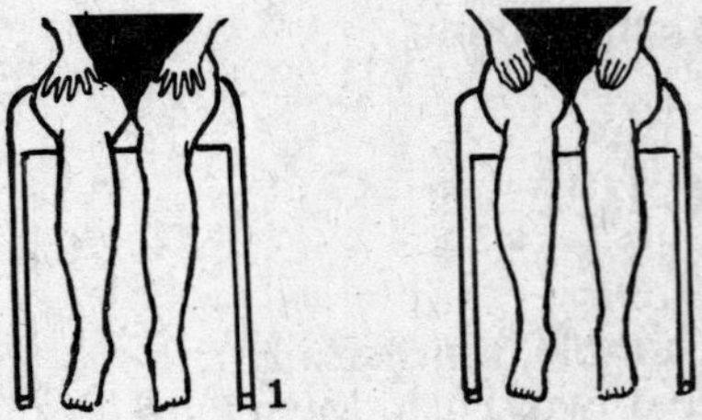

hem raiser

stiff knee

1 Sit on a chair or stool.

2 With back straight, stretch out left leg really tightly, raising the foot off the floor.

3 Lower the leg.

4 With back straight, stretch out right leg really tightly, raising the foot off the floor.

5 Lower the leg.

Do exercise eight to 10 times.

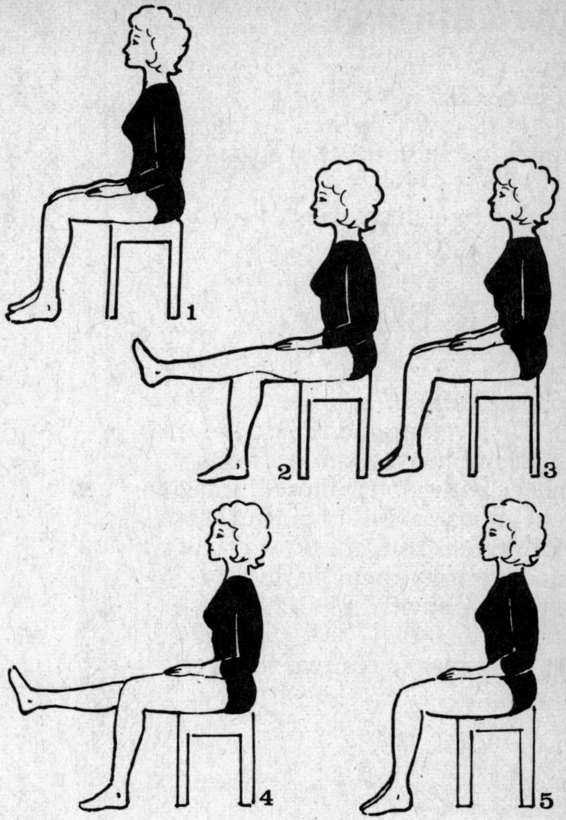

scarf trick

toning thickening ankles and strengthening them

1 Stand with bare feet. Spread the edge of a silk or similar, slippery scarf under the toes. Pull scarf under feet by pulling back toes . . .

2 . . . and stretching them again.

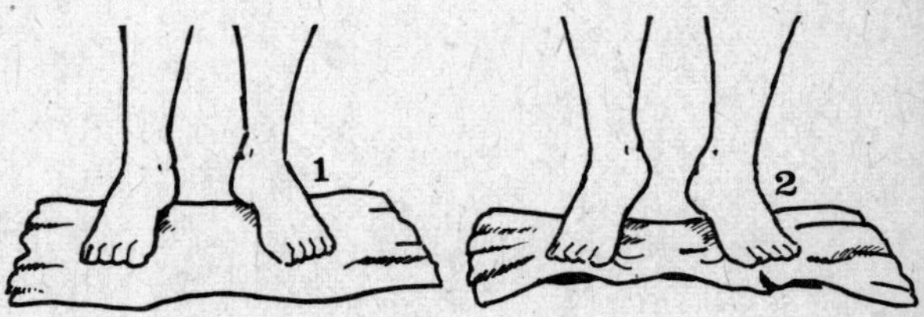

one chin less

chinline and neck toning
1 Push lower lip well up over upper lip. Push up chin aggressively.

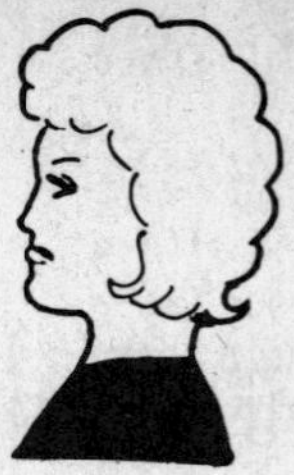

Do five to eight pushes.

bubble blower

nose-to-mouth lines
1 Do as many models do before a photographic session: puff out cheeks with mouth closed. Imagine your mouth is full of air bubbles. More them from cheek to cheek, concentrating them behind the upper and lower lips.

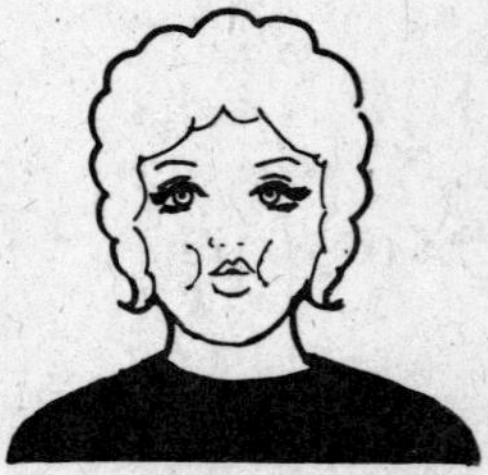

Do the exercise for two to three minutes.

FOR MEN AND WOMEN

a better way to stand

A slack stance throws body out of true. It puts strain on back, hunches shoulders, pushes muscles into the wrong position which invites flab.

Bad posture is an early ager. Round shoulders, protruding seat and stomach are all signs that posture-improving movements could help.

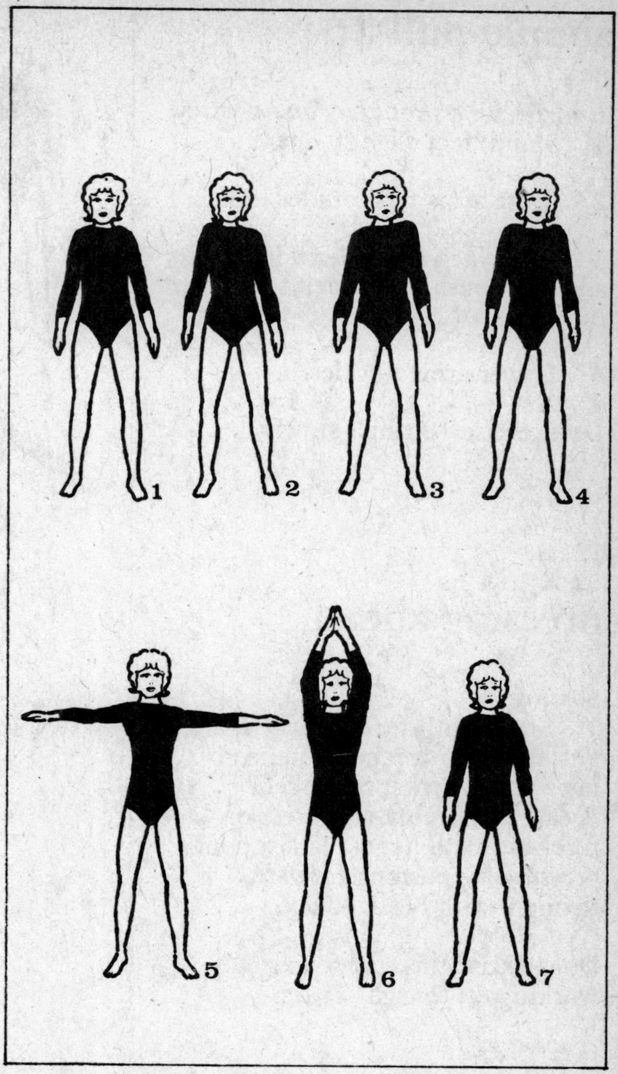

fledgling

1 Stand, feet a little apart, arms loosely at sides.

2 Circle right shoulder backwards twice.

3 Circle left shoulder backwards twice.

4 Circle both shoulders.

5 Raise arms out.

6 Put up arms to meet above head, and at the same time rise on toes.

7 Lower down on to heels as arms lower to sides again.

Do whole movement three times, working up to eight.

simple pull up

straightening shoulders and posture

1 Stand, feet slightly apart.

2 Raise arms to shoulder level.

3 Push back from shoulders once, and then push arms back to straight out position.

4 Lower arms to sides.

Do exercise 10 times slowly.

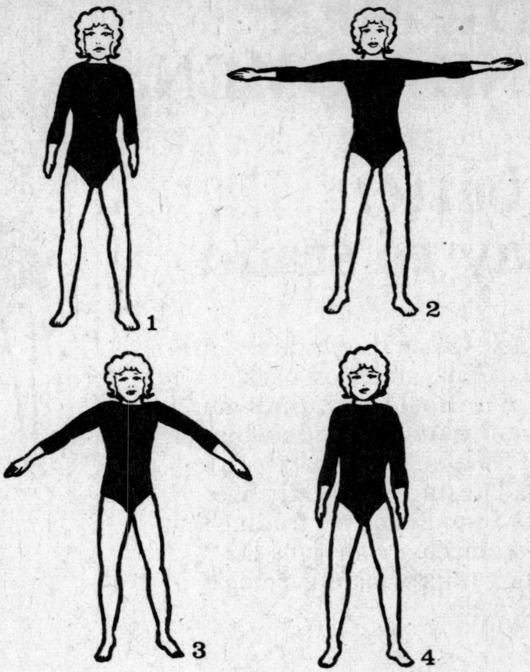

pressing ahead

posture

1 Stand with feet slightly apart. Put hands on forehead, palms inwards, fingers interlocked. Breathe in deeply and press on forehead with hands. Resist hand pressure by pushing forward strongly with head. Relax.

Do exercise three or four times, working up to eight or ten.

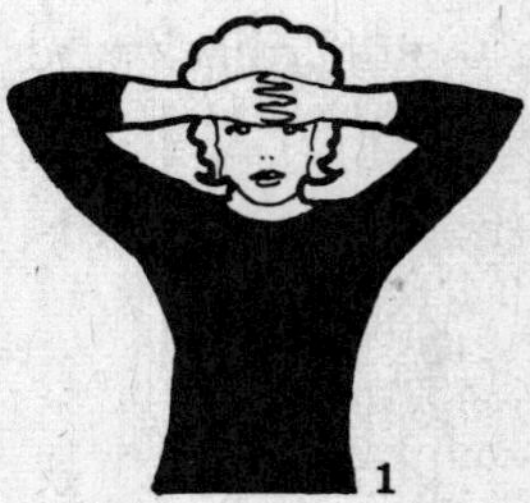

on the hop

1 Stand with feet together, arms at sides.

2 Taking the weight on the left foot, pull right foot up leg, with right knee pointing to right.

3 Tuck right foot into left thigh, as far up as you can. (You may need to hold on to something solid with right hand, while pulling up foot with left hand, until you get your balance.)

4 Stand straight, and raise arms outwards and up to meet, palm to palm, prayerwise above the head.

5 Lower arms.

6 Slowly lower leg.

7 With weight on right foot, pull left foot up let, left knee pointing leftwards. Tuck left foot into right thigh, as far up as you can go.

8 Stand straight, and raise arms outwards and up to meet above head, as before.

9 Slowly lower leg.

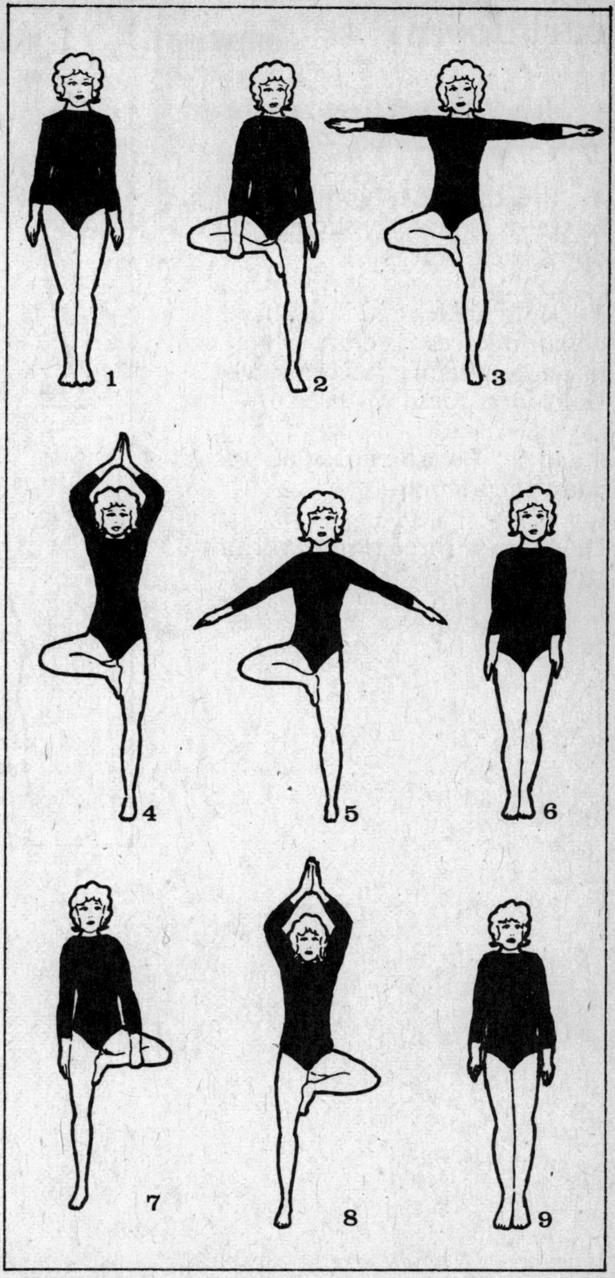

curl down

1 Stand straight, feet together, arms at sides. Breathe in.

2 Breathe out as you bend forwards from *hips,* sliding hands down back of legs.

3 Hold ankles and bring head down to knees (as close as you can manage), keeping knees straight. Hold for a count of three.

4 and 5 Breathe in as you uncurl and straighten up.

Do exercise three times, working up to 10.

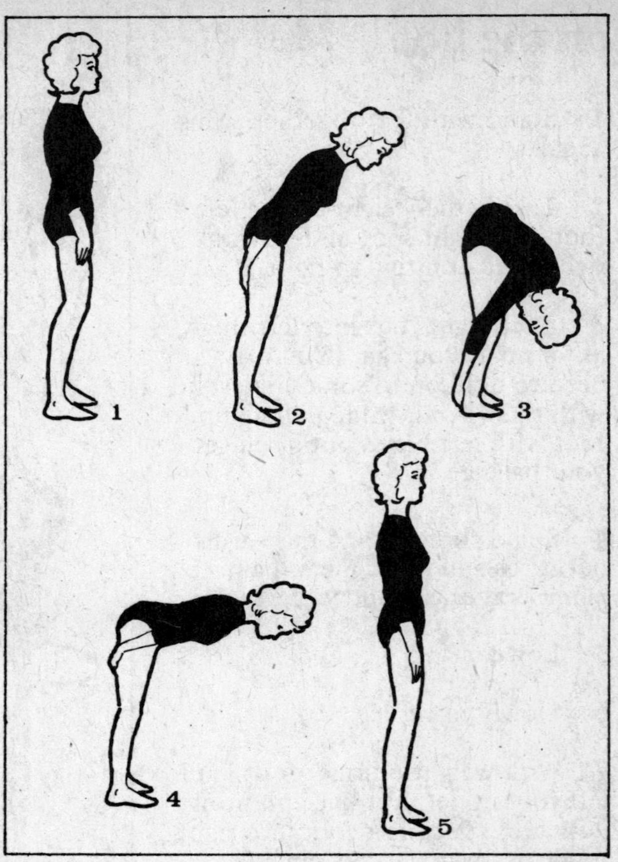

hedgehog

1 Kneel, with toes turned in.

2 Sit back on heels, wrapping hands round heels. Breathe in.

3 Breathe out, keeping a firm hold on heels as you bend forward, so you are pushing forward on floor with head. Keep feet on floor. Count a slow three.

4 Breathe in as you straighten up to sit back on heels again.

Do exercise three times, increasing to 10.

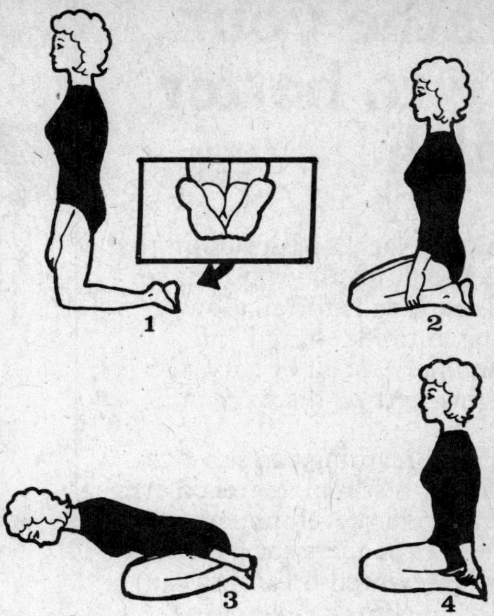

bridge

1 Lay on floor, hands under thighs, palms down.

2 Taking weight on forearms, arch back and rest top of head on mat with neck stretched. Hold for a slow count of three.

3 Relax slowly to starting position.

Do exercise three times, up to 10.

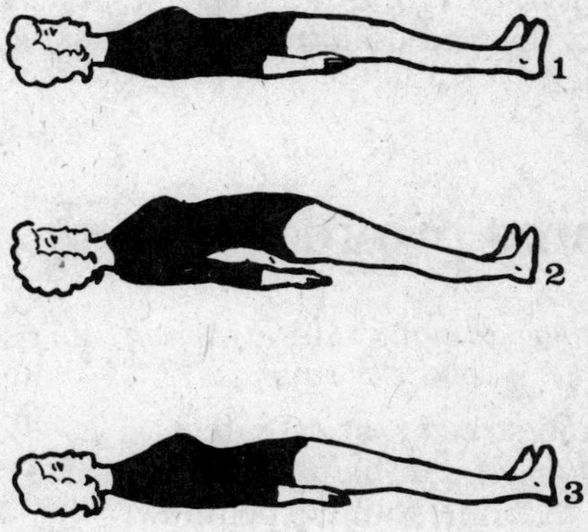

breathe your way to better health

Breathing is such a basic action that few people think about it. But so often breathing is too shallow, resulting in tiredness and sluggishness. And all because the body's not getting the oxygen it needs.

Correct breathing can serve several uses – stimulate, relax, even aid in muscular development (see the Chest Expanders for men in this section). Measured breathing can also lend impetus to exercises which strengthens their effect.

The bonus to the movements here is that they make you think about breathing well which means you may look (goodbye sallowness) and feel (up and doing) much healthier.

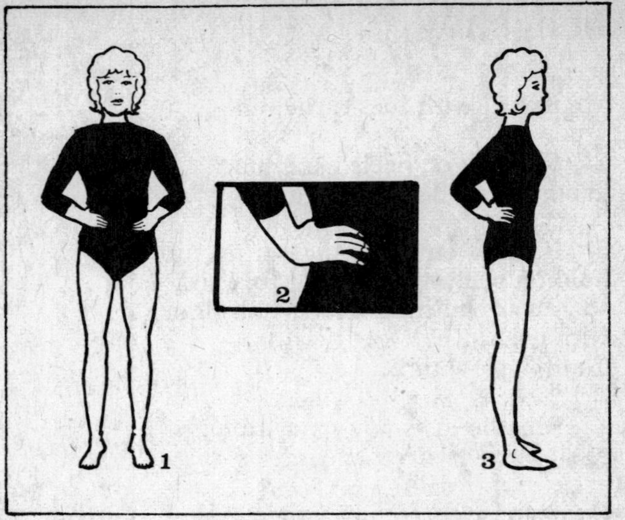

pushing proud

breathing   *bulging sides of trunk, shoulder to waist*

1 Stand straight, at ease, feet slightly apart. Put hands on waist, fingers in front, thumbs behind.

2 Breathe in deeply, lifting chest really high. Press hands hard against hips all the time you are breathing in.

3 Breathe out and relax.

Do the exercise three or four times to begin, working up to eight or 10.

way up, way down

breathing
1 Stand, feet slightly apart, arms at sides.

2 *Breathe in* as you raise arms above head.

3 Then *breathe out* as arms lower and you bend, trying to touch knees with head and clasp ankles.

4 *Breathe in* as you unfurl and raise arms above head again. Now bend down again, trying to touch knees with head and clasp ankles.

Do the whole movement five times, working up to 10. Keep continuous and flowing.

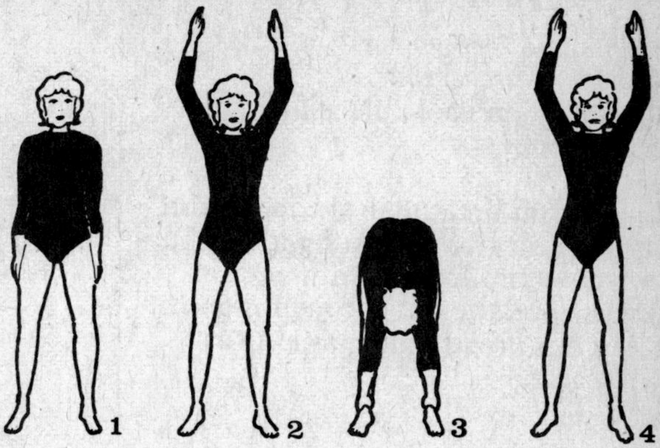

chest expander, one

(for men) breathing
1 Lying on your back, draw up knees and rest hands over lower part of lungs.

2 Breathe in through nose and push stomach out against hands.

3 As you breathe out, stomach draws in. Make out breath last as long as you can.

Do three in-out breaths, working up to 10.

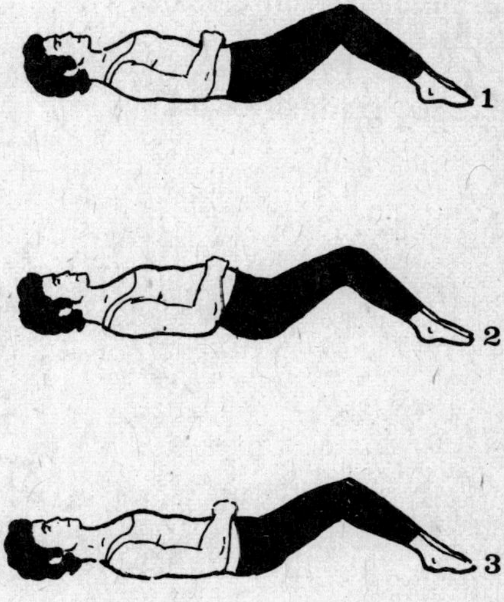

chest expander, two

(for men) breathing
1 Lying on back, place hands at sides of ribs.

2 As you breathe in through nose, try to push ribs against hands. (The power comes from breath and lungs.) Breathe out through mouth. Keep out-breath going as long as you can.

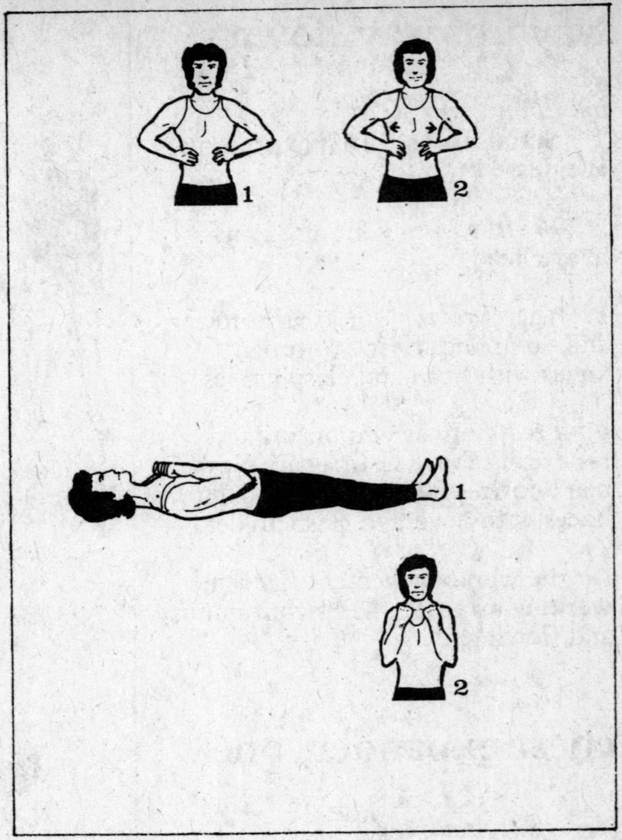

chest expander, three

(for men)
1 and 2 Lay down, bending elbows and resting hands, clenched into fists, on collar bones. Breathe in – a long breath through the nose. Breathe out in short, sharp, hard breaths.

Do three times, gradually working up to 10.

'cleansing' breath, one

yoga origins, and helps circulation, alertness

1 Stand straight, with feet together and arms at sides.

2 *Breathe in* deeply through nose and raise arms slowly forwards and up above head.

3 With arms up, hold breath for 'one and . . .'

4 On count of 'two', breathe out through mouth with a loud, hard breath and let trunk drop forwards, arms swinging down and loose.

Straighten up and go into the exercise again. Do it rhythmically four or five times, working up to seven.

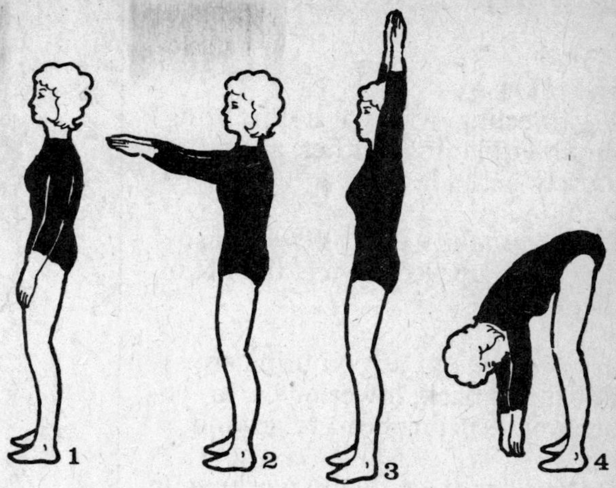

'cleansing' breath, two

yoga origins

1 Sit cross-legged, with hands resting on knees. Breathe in long and deeply through both nostrils.

2 Pull in stomach and diaphragm muscles sharply, so that air is forced out of nose fast.

Repeat this straight away four more times. Add another set of five long in-breaths, short, sharp out-breaths as you grow used to it. Then another set. Allow a minute of normal breathing between sets.

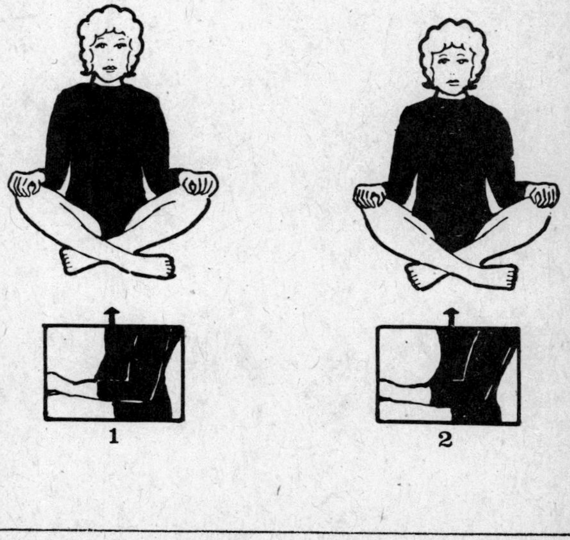

salaam

breathing

1 Kneeling, with chest out, bring shoulder blades together, arms loosely behind.

2 *Breathe in* as you slowly raise arms high up. Really feel the lift in diaphragm.

3 *Breathe out* as you bring arms down and back, lowering on to heels and curling head to ground.

Do five times, gradually working up to 15.

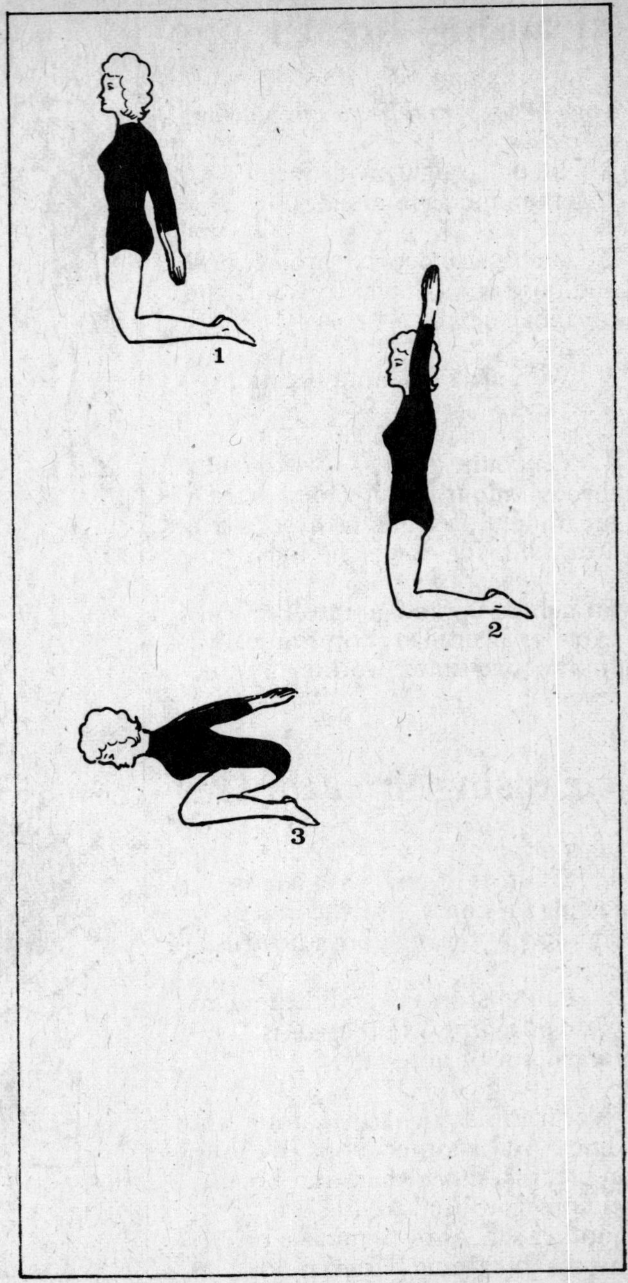

windmills

breathing
1 Lay down, with feet against a wall and arms at sides.

2 to 4 *Breathe in* as you raise arms slowly up in front of you, then down to above head.

5 and 6 *Breathe out* as you lower arms sideways to sides.

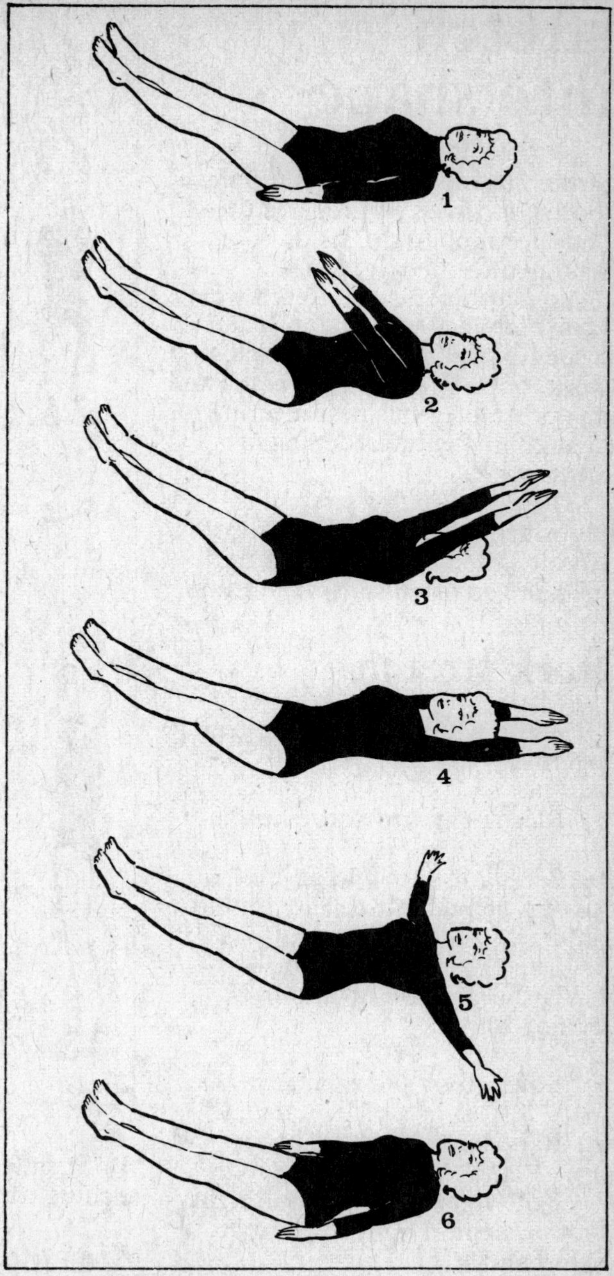

stretch into shape

Stretching makes muscles supple, loosens stiffness. It prepares the body for mobility. Cats do it on waking up – people, too.

You automatically stretch when your body has been in 'muscular suspense', i.e. hunched over close work, or body movement restricted in a protracted business meeting, or bent coping with gardening or housework.

The right kind of stretching movements keeps the back flexible. And it's the back that takes the load and so often shows the strain.

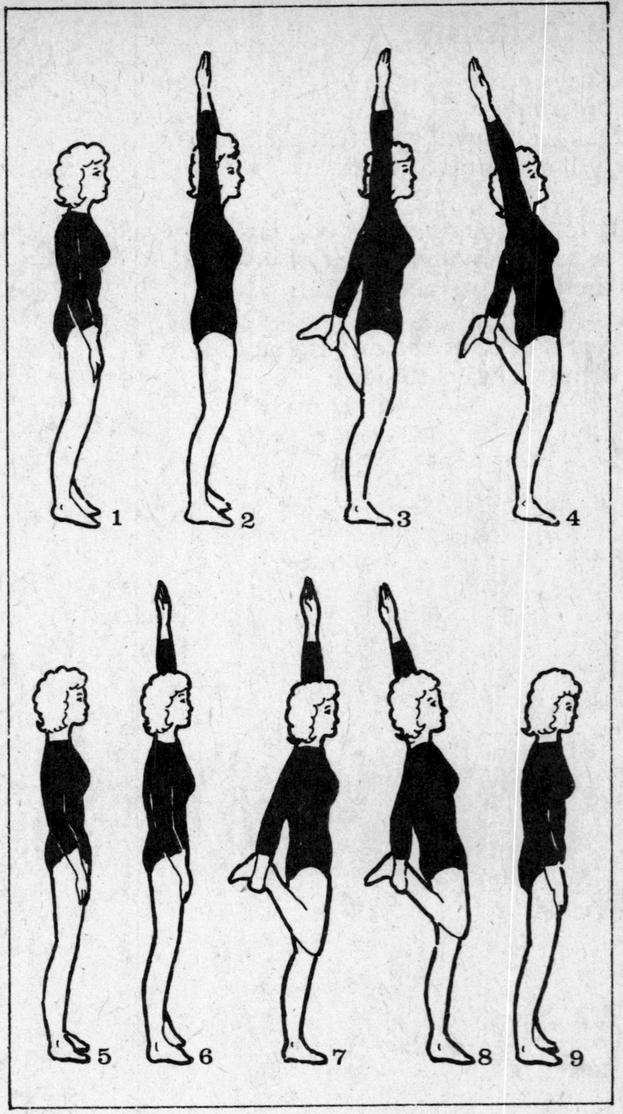

stork stretch

1 Stand with arms at sides, feet together.

2 Raise right arm above head.

3 Bend left knee and pull left foot up behind left thigh with left hand.

4 Push right arm up and back, arching trunk.

5 Lower foot and then arm.

6 Raise left arm above head.

7 Bend right knee and pull right foot up behind right thigh with right hand.

8 Push left arm right up and back, arching trunk.

9 Lower foot and then arm.

cloud catcher

stretching

1 Stand, feet comfortably apart, arms at sides, a little back from body.

2 Raise arms slowly sideways.

3 Interlock fingers above head, turn palms upwards and stretch as high as you can from waist.

4 Separate hands, lower arms sideways.

Breathe in going up. Breathe out coming down. Do exercise three times working up to 10.

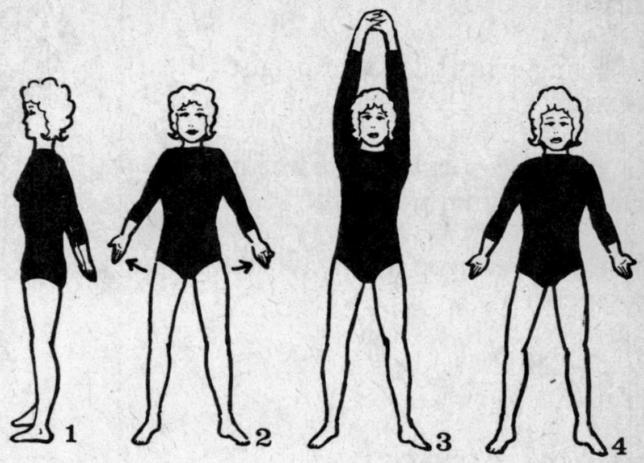

each way stretch

stretching

1 Stand, feet comfortably apart, arms at sides, a little back from the body.

2 Breathe in as arms go up.

3 Interlock fingers and hold arms upwards, elbows a little relaxed.

4 Slowly bend to left.

Continued overleaf

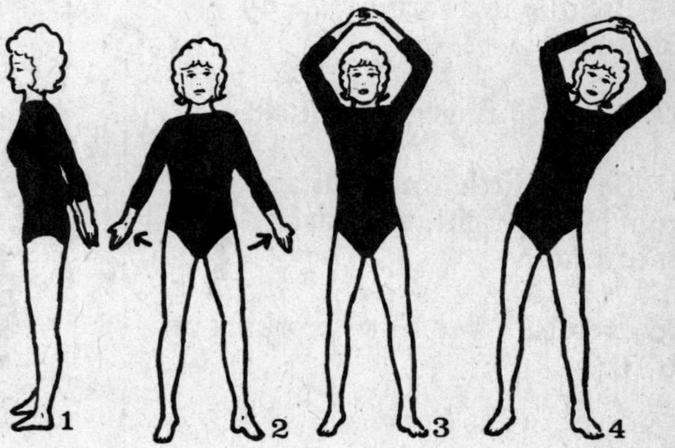

5 Bend to right, holding in drawn breath.

6 Bring arms back to upright position.

7 Breathe out, while lowering arms to original position.

Do exercise three times, working up to seven.

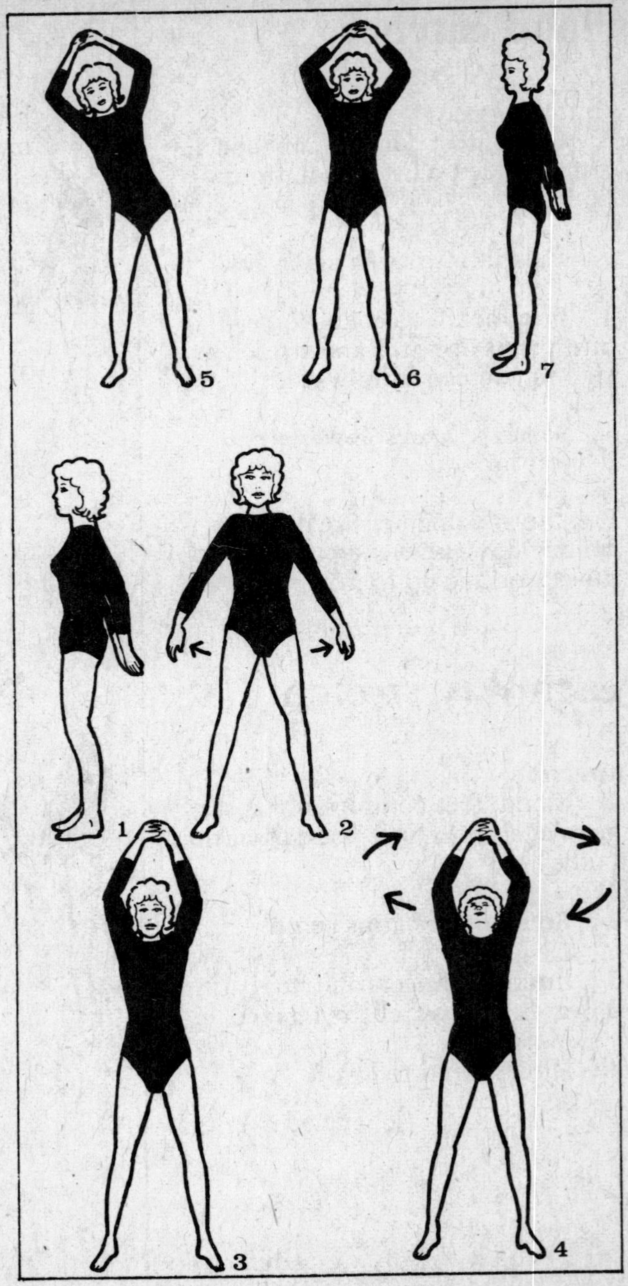

swivel stretch

1 Stand, feet comfortably apart, arms at sides, a little back from body.

2 Breathe in as arms raise up sideways . . .

3 . . . until fingers interlock.

4 Bend a little forwards and circle from hips – right, then back, left and front.

Do exercise three times working up to 10.

rocking cradle

stretching

1 Sit, left leg straight out in front, right knee bent, arms wrapped round bent knee, back straight.

2 Slowly curl trunk over bent knee, vertebra by vertebra, until head is resting on it.

3 Roll back in this position using bent knee as leverage.

4 Roll back to starting position.

5 Slowly straighten trunk.

Do this five times.

6 Now sit with the right leg straight, and left leg bent at knee, with arms wrapped around bent knee. Keep back straight.

7 Slowly curl trunk over bent knee until head is resting on it.

8 Roll back in this position, using bent knee as leverage.

9 Roll back to starting position.

10 Slowly straighten trunk.

Do this five times.

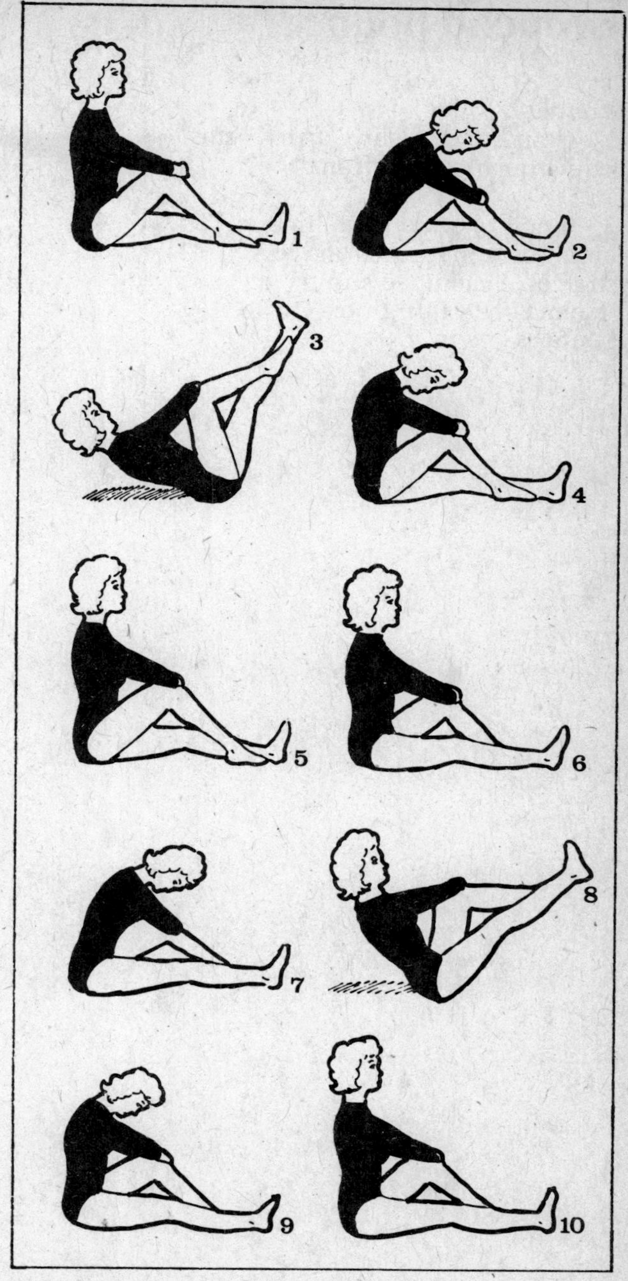

Groucho bounce

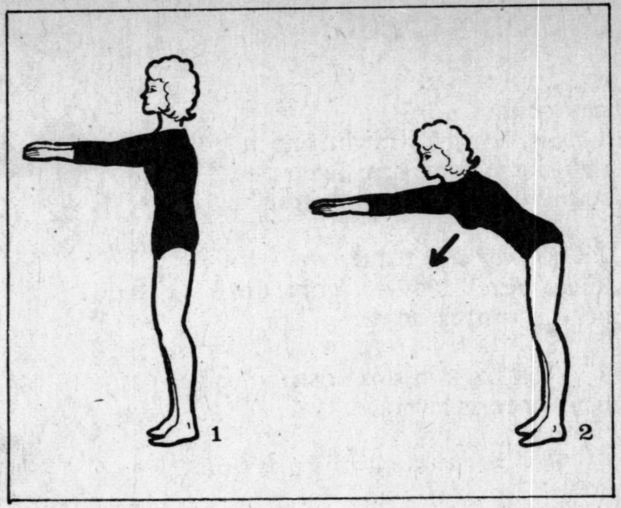

stretching

1 Stand, feet slightly apart, arms held straight out in front.

2 Bend forward from hips and hold position – arms and legs straight, head up – and try to 'bounce' chest on floor. Do 15 bounces.

his and hers isometrics

Exercises fall into two groups: isotonics and isometrics. Most of the exercises in this book are isotonic – where movement is fairly free. These exercises not only tone muscles in a specific area but stimulate circulation and aid in consuming calories which helps reduce fat.

Isometrics have a more concentrated effect. Their action is to present resistance to movement. Complete dedication to them builds a strong-muscled Mr Universe. In moderation they'll strengthen weak and disused muscles. They, too, check sag, but perhaps their prime function is to reduce fatigue in the use of a muscle. For example: anyone desk-bound may be prone to aches in the upper back from leaning over close work. Someone new to standing for long periods will find legs soon tire. Lifting and raising arms wearies untrained arms and shoulder muscles.

Isometrics are also useful where space and circumstances don't allow for lots of movement. *The following exercises are suitable for both men and women.* More are featured for men in the Businessman's Keep Fit Format.

one for the mantelshelf

shoulders, upper back

1 With feet well apart, press palms down on a hard surface at shoulder level. Do three or four presses, three or four times. Work up to 10 times three or four.

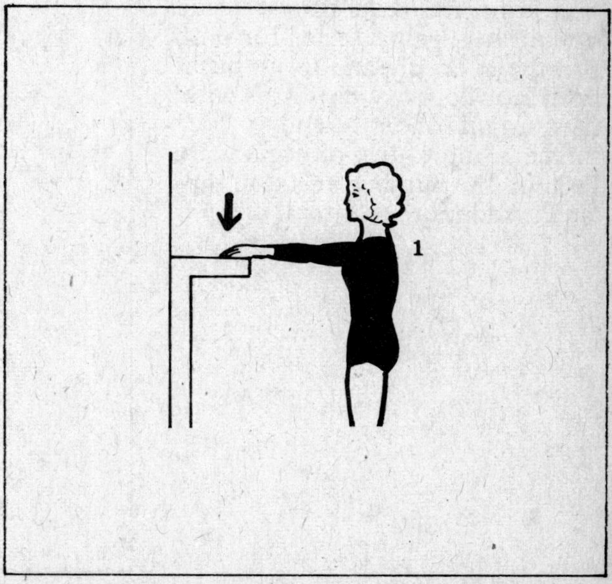

hand in hand

arms and shoulders

1 Standing or sitting, with arms behind back, press fist of right hand into cupped left hand. Really resist, with two or three pushes.

2 Press left fist into cupped right hand, again resisting with two or three pushes.

Do whole movement three times, working up to 10 times.

angel wings

upper arms

1 Stand in a doorway, feet a little apart. Grip hands into fists and raise arms. Rest fists against insides of doorway, palms facing forwards. Breathe in deeply and try to push insides of doorway outwards with fists. Count 'one, two and three . . .' up to five to begin with. Push on the number, relax on the 'and'. Add more to a total of 15.

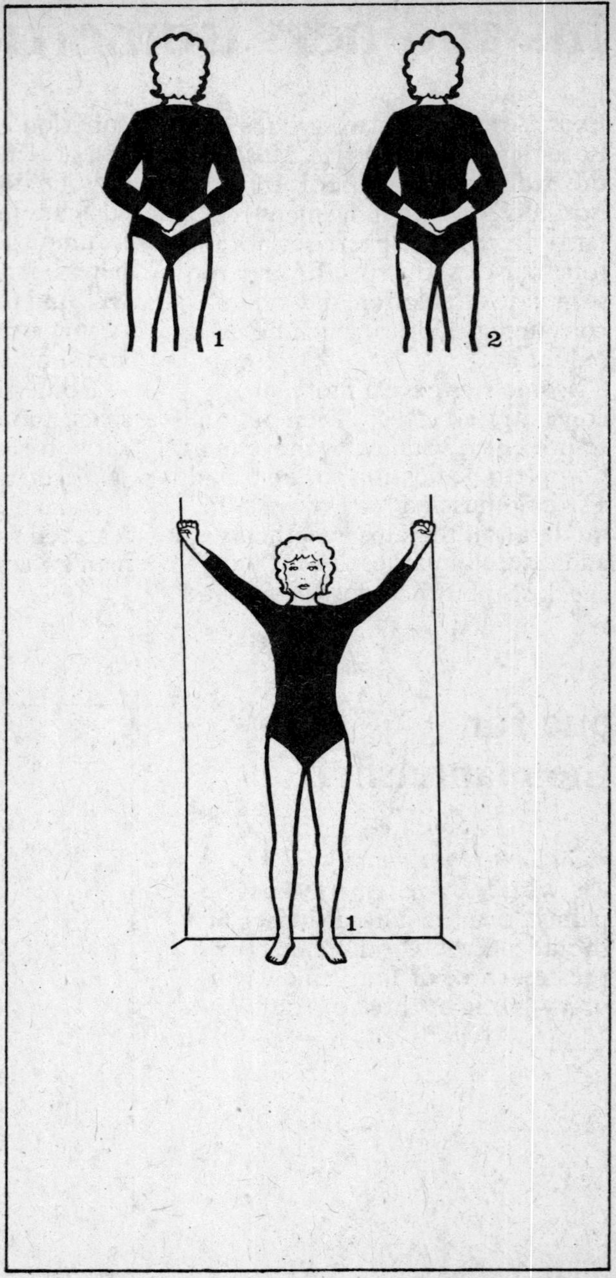

big push

upper arms

1 Stand facing wall, feet about 12 inches away. Raise arms and place heels of hands against wall at eye level. Press hard against wall with heels of hands. Count 'one and two and . . .' up to five, pressing on the numbers, relaxing on 'and'. Work up to 15.

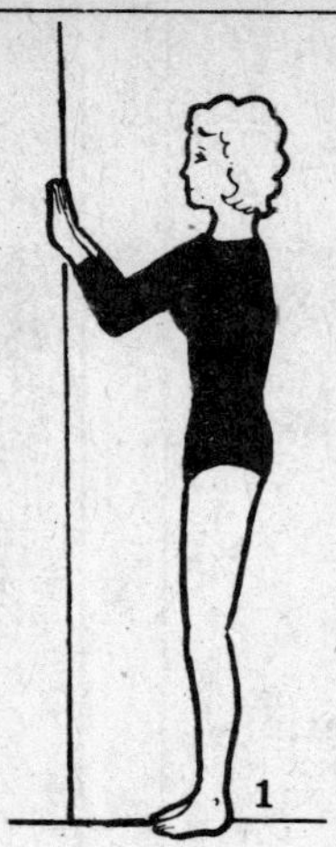

see-saw

strengthening wrists

1 Sit down at table or desk, resting on elbows and holding hands as if praying.

2 Raise left elbow so that left hand can go with right hand as you push it back towards right shoulder. Now begin to apply pressure as you try to straighten right wrist, while left resists for about a minute.

3 Return to initial position.

4 Raise right elbow, so that right hand can go with left hand, as you try to push it back towards the left shoulder.

Do exercise two or three times with each hand, working up gradually to eight or 10.

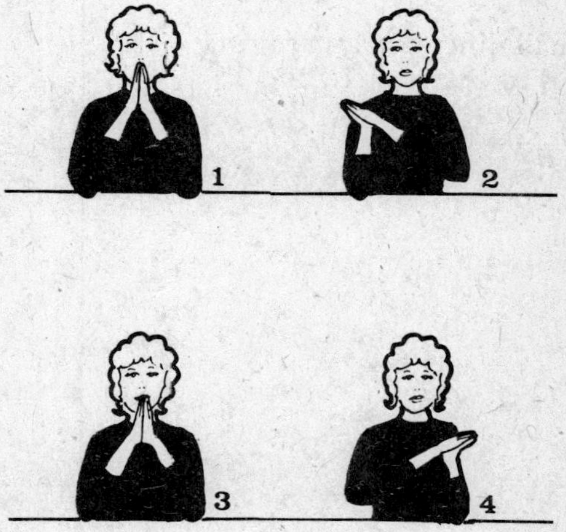

ballet stretch

sides of midriff and waist

1 Stand, right side to a wall, feet together, about 18 inches away.

2 Raise left arm up and over head to place palm against wall. Push hand against wall.

3 Relax.

4 Stand with left side to the wall, 18 inches away.

5 Raise right arm up and over head to place palm against wall. Push hand against wall. Relax.

Gradually increase arm-raising-presses to between 10 and 15.

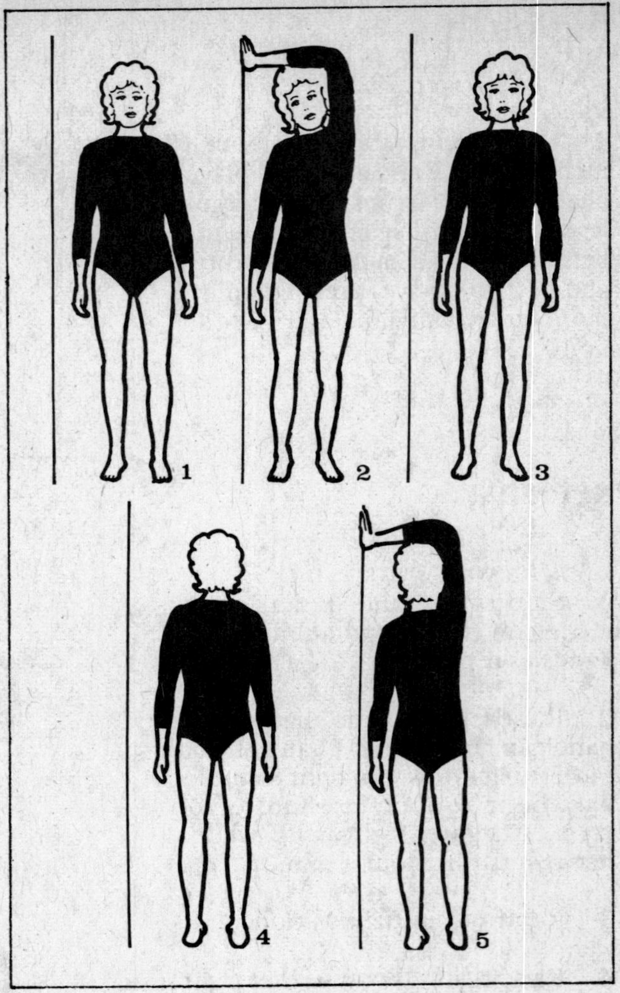

indignant sergeant major

midriff

1 Stand, feet slightly apart, hands on hips.

2 Breathe in long and deeply, lifting chest, and press down with hands as hard as you can. Keep back straight. Relax.

Do five times, working up to 15. Slowly and forcefully.

gravity – for and against

waist and stomach

1 Sit on floor, legs straight out.

2 Bend forwards, resting hands just below knees. Push down with hands, push up with legs to resist hands.

Do exercise eight times, working up to 15.

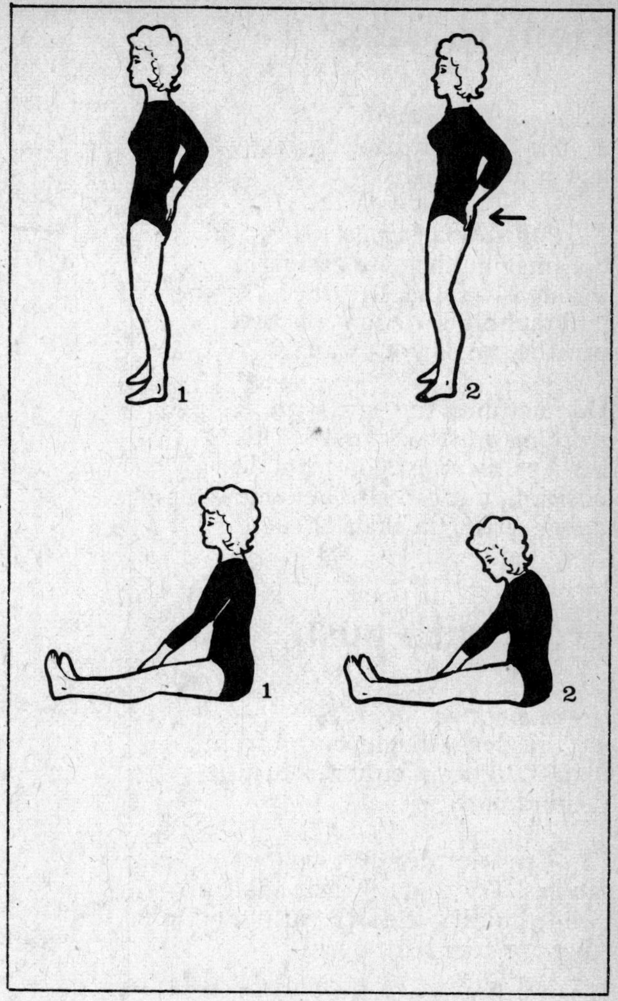

front to back

waist and stomach
1 Sit on floor, back against wall, legs straight out.

2 Pull stomach muscles in, and up. Imagine they are getting through to spine. Breathe in as you pull in, hold for count of three, breathe out as you relax.

Do five times to begin with, working up slowly to 15. This is perhaps the most comfortable position, but can also be done lying down, sitting in chair or standing.

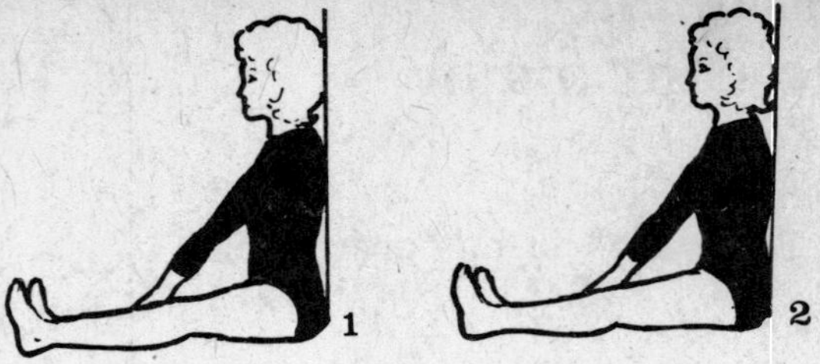

cross with push

front and back of thighs
1 Sit, legs straight out in front, hands on floor, either side, just behind body.

2 Cross left leg over right at ankles. Try to push right ankle up while holding it down with left. Do three or four hard pushes.

3 Again, put legs out straight.

4 Cross right leg over left at ankles. Try to push ankle up while holding it down with right.

Work up to 10 or 12 with each leg.

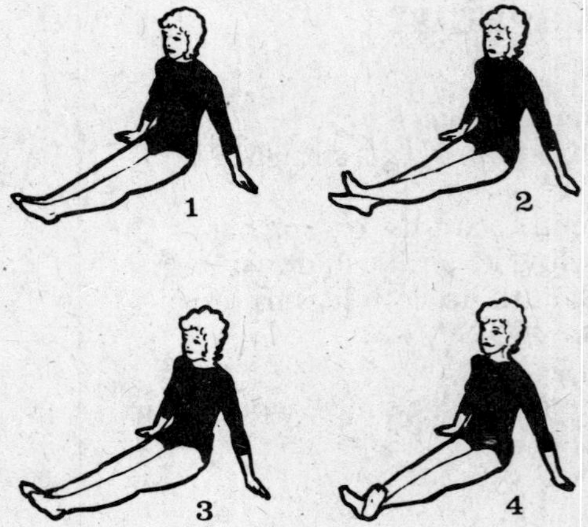

push in, push out

inside thighs

1 Sit with back straight, legs straight out together, place left hand against outside of left knee, and right hand outside of right knee. Push hands inwards, trying to push legs wide against resistance of hands.

Do exercise eight or 10 times, working up to 20.

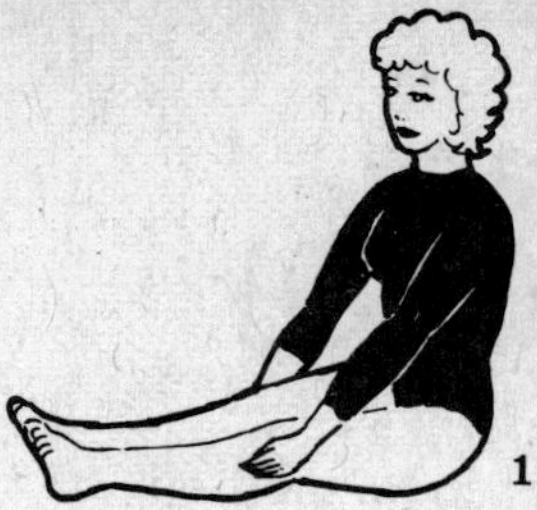

1

leg puller

outside thighs

1 Sit with legs out straight. Cross ankles. Keep firmly crossed while trying to pull them apart.

Do five times, gradually working up to 20.

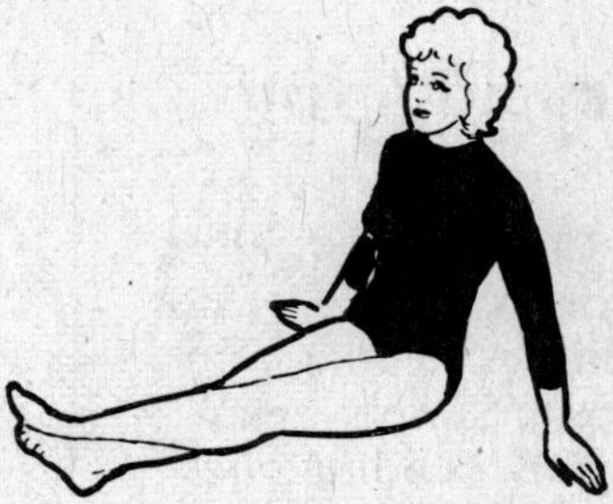

1

on your toes

calves

1 Sit, legs straight out in front, hands resting on floor at either side behind body for support.

2 Place ball of right foot against tops of toes of left foot. Press and relax 10 times.

3 Place ball of left foot against tops of toes of right foot. Press and relax 10 times.

Work up to 20 times with each foot.

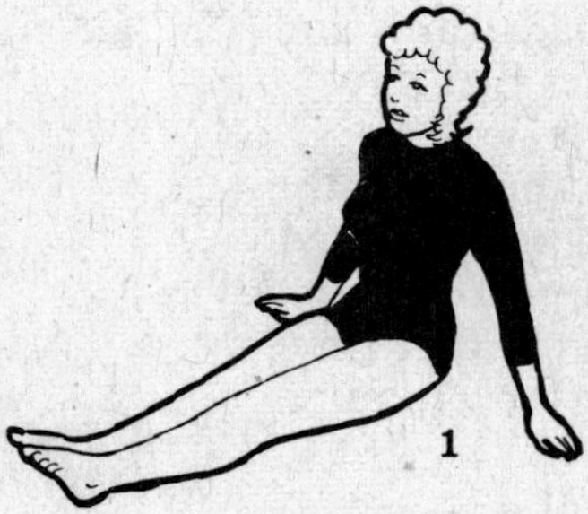

1

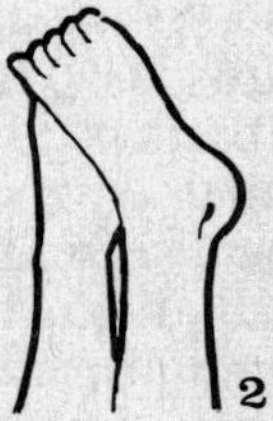

2

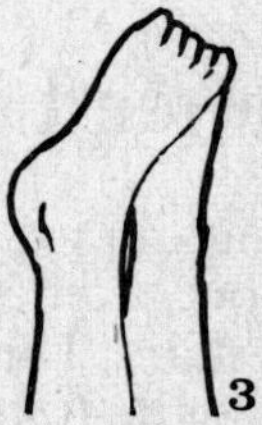

3

jogging – preliminary and advanced

Popular in the States and a method approved here. It's really a modified form of running. It's more vigorous than you'd think until you try doing it and should be taken easily at first.

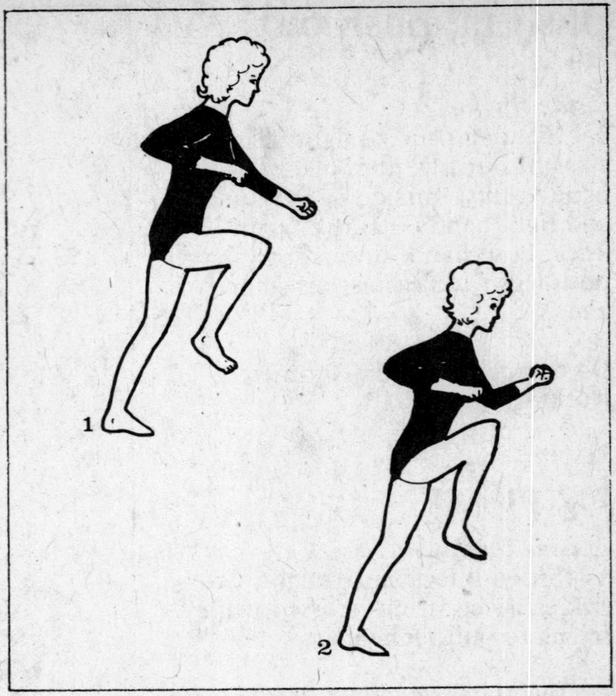

preliminary jogging

1 A good way to start, especially if you're out of condition and/or not used to exercising, is to do a kind of drum-majorette. Simply mark time on the spot by bending one knee and raising it as high as you can – then the other. Foot of straight leg stays firmly on the ground. Swing arms backwards and forwards. Two minutes first day; three the next, five the next.

Fourth day: start running on the spot but keep lifting knee or raised leg really high. You'll probably find half a minute enough the first time. Next day you can try for a minute.

advanced jogging

2 You can jog on the spot or on the move, you can also run up and down stairs. The idea is gradually to increase the *time* time you spend jogging; the *distance* – if you're able to run about freely, and the *number of times* you raise each leg during your jogging sessions.

It tends to be easier for men than for women, and it's considered that if a woman can manage two or three minutes at one time she's above average. But when did that ever stop anyone?

FOR MEN
businessman's keep fit format

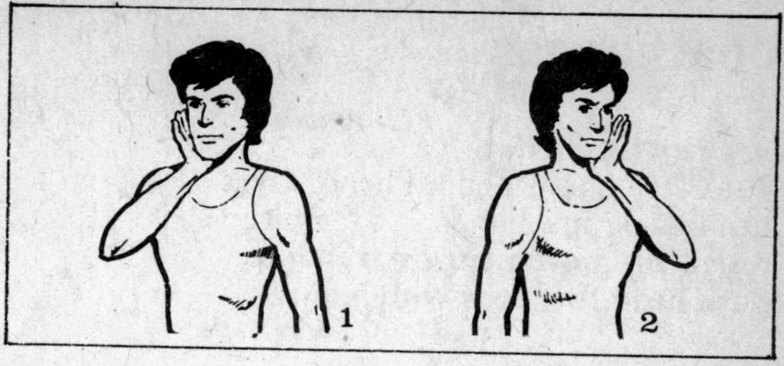

These are all isometric movements – static exercises where muscles contract without the joints moving. This means they can be carried out within a confined space – such as office, car (when not driving of course).

The following are all designed to be done from a sitting position, so they're specially convenient. They can be practised individually to tone specific areas but ideally the whole 10 should be run through. The more effort that goes into them, the better they build up muscle. 'Should be done to an intensity where muscles shake with the effort' says our physiotherapist, if you're aiming to body-build.

'The more repetitions you can build up, the more successful you will be in increasing power and muscle bulk.'

Useful for the not-so-young – practised from a comfortable chair – but they should take the movements more easily at first.

uppercut

chinline and neck

1 Head turned slightly to left, lift chin with heel of hand, fingers splayed. Press down hard *on* hand while pushing up hard *with* hand.

2 Repeat movement with right hand, head turned slightly to right.

face bracer

This is the same exercise as in 'switching off the pressure' (page 131). Clench face muscles, squeeze up eyes, bare teeth, and concertina nose. Pull as many expressions as you can.

coathanger

neck and shoulders
1 Clasp hands behind head. Press head back into hands. At same time resist this movement by trying to push head forwards with hands.

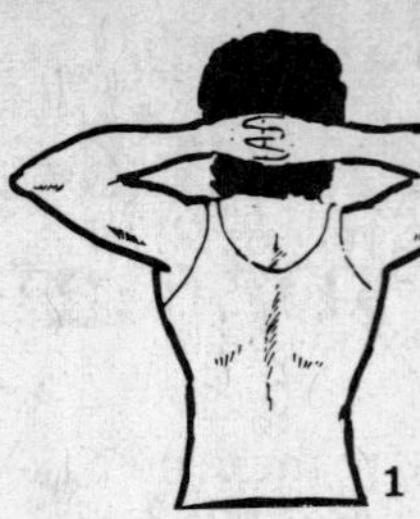

big pusher

chest and arm muscles
1 With arms bent at shoulder level in front, link fingers and place heels of hands together. Lift elbows and press heels of hands hard together as though you were trying to crack a nut between them.

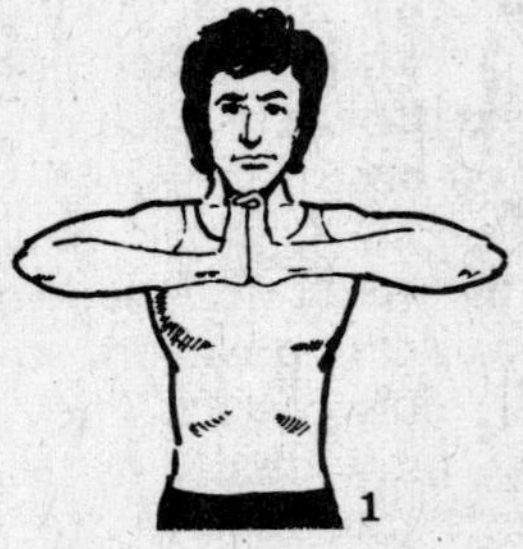

a firm front

for stomach
1 Sit in a chair with a firm back.

2 Press small of back hard into chair. The back is kept straight and flat against back of chair. Try to get lower ribs to meet top of pelvis. Stomach muscles should tense as if anticipating a blow.

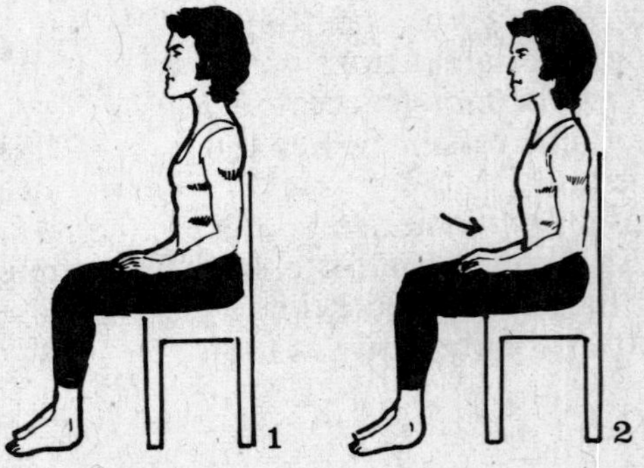

floor shaker

buttocks
1 Sit with feet together, flat on floor. Try to push floor away from you as hard as you can with feet.

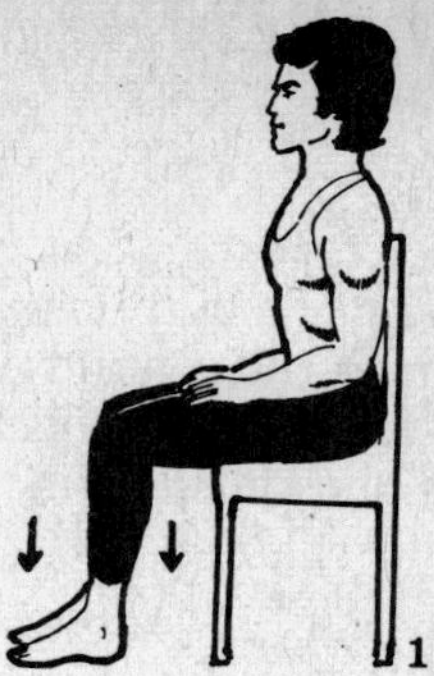

1

thigh quaker

thighs
1 Sit with legs straight out and together. Contract thigh muscles by straightening knees as hard as you can.

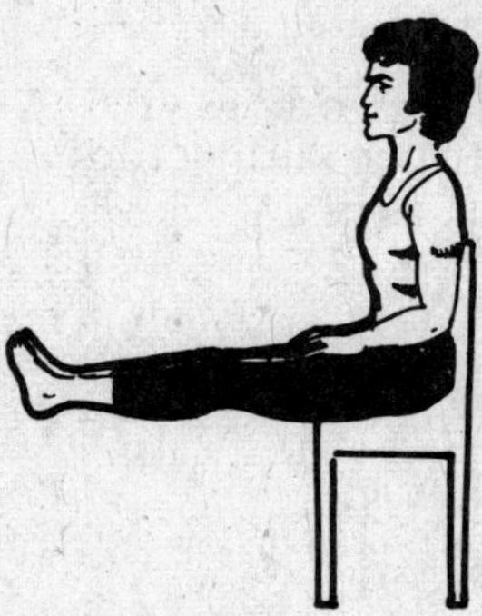

1

shin hardener

shins
1 Sit with legs together, heels firmly on floor, and pull toes up hard towards you as if trying to make toes meet shins.

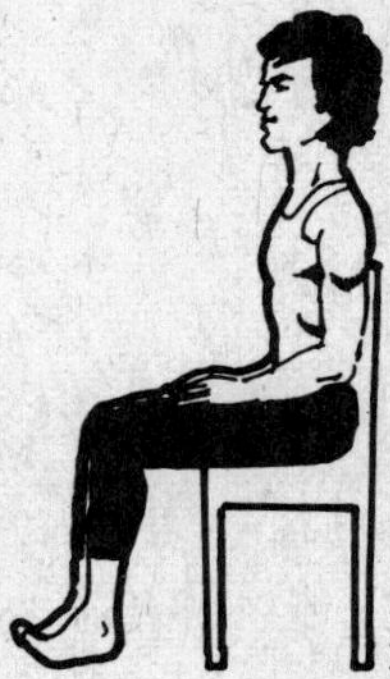

1

calf toughener

calves
1 Sit with feet together, flat on ground, and lift heels by pressing them up hard into the ground with the ball of the foot. Keep balls of feet on ground and press them down hard.

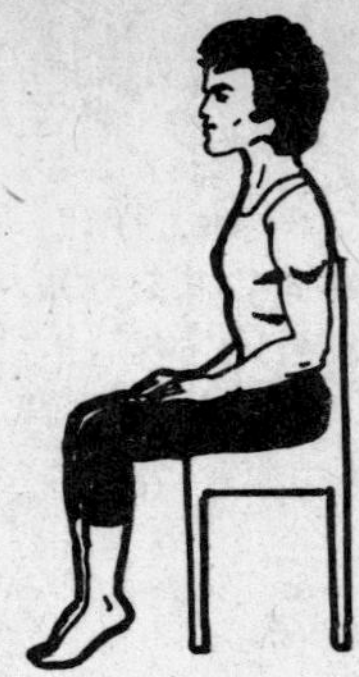

1

extreme measures

hands and feet
1 Clench fists as tightly as you can, at the same time curling toes under hard.

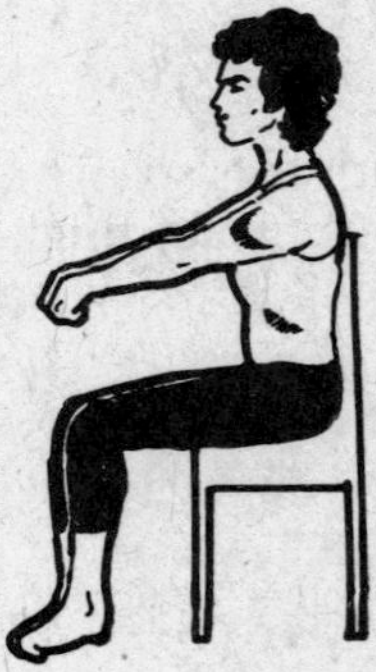

1

fat fighters and power drivers (men only)

Those marked ● are planned in progressions. Power – and body building – is effected by first practising the easier movements. As the muscles become accustomed to these, they're built up to several 'repeats'. After this, you move on to the tougher movements of the routine.

Just following the first half of any of the routines keeps the body toned, and this could be a sufficient goal for the not-so-young and the fat prone.

Once you reach the final movement you're really body-building.

four progression programmes

Progression plan: In each ● routine, start by practising movement number 1 *three* times. Increase each day until you're doing it ten times.

Keep up these ten repetitions but add movement number 2. Just *once* at first, gradually increasing to ten.

When you've reached twenty times – i.e. movements 1 and 2 ten times each, drop 1 altogether, and add the third movement – just *once* the first day, increasing by one each day until you're doing it ten times.

Again – at twenty times – ten times for the second and ten times for the third, you drop the second and add the fourth – *once* to begin with, increasing each day up to ten.

Finally, you're practising movements 3 and 4, ten times each, every day. Keep a steady rhythm. Aim to increase speed.

With the other exercises, weights mentioned can be training weights from sports shops, cans of food, or very stout bags holding potatoes, sawdust, sand or earth.

• for big chest

1 Get down on all fours, touch nose to ground, taking weight on hands. Lift head up. Relax.

2 Repeat movement, first with right leg kneeling and left leg straight. Lift head as you complete movement with each leg.

3 Repeat movement, with both legs out straight. Head down, then up.

4 Repeat movement, this time with feet on a low stool. Head down, then up.

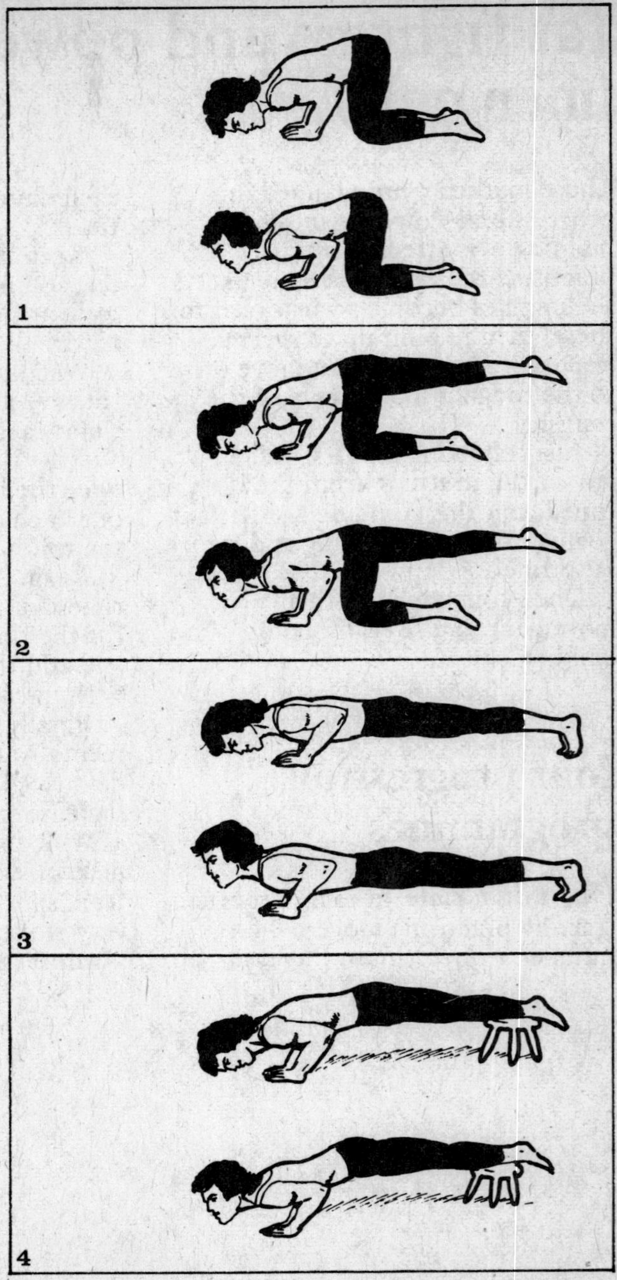

• for tailoring diaphragm

1 Lie on back, with arms outstretched, knees bent and feet flat on floor. Swing knees to touch floor on one side, then swing to the other side. Keep knees together.

2 Repeat movement, but keep the right leg straight, then the left leg straight. Foot of bent leg against knee of straight leg.

3 Still swinging side to side, knees bent and feet off the floor.

4 Repeat movement, but keep both legs together.

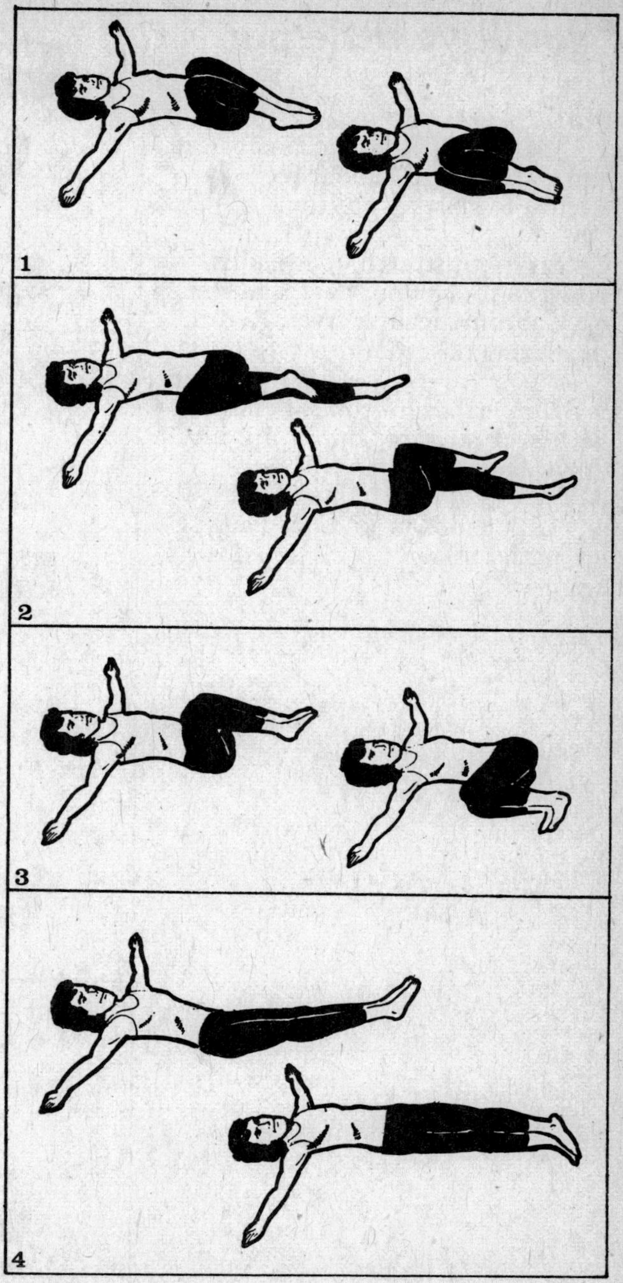

• goodbye little pot

stomach strengthener

1 Lie flat on your back. Lift head and shoulders to look at feet. Return to starting position.

2 Sit up to stretch your hands down to touch your toes, and the back automatically curves. Return to starting position.

3 Link hands in front of chest, with back straight, and sit up. Lie down again.

4 Link hands behind head and sit up, with a straight back. Lie down again.

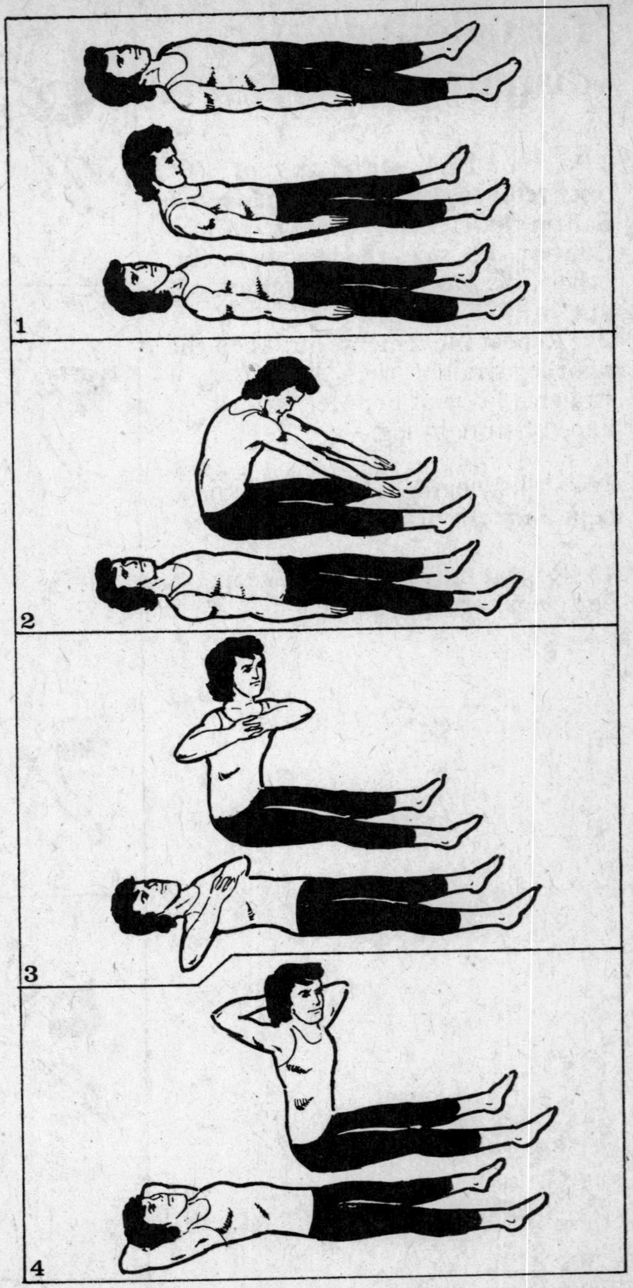

• trim back

back strengthener, seat tautener

1 Lie down facing floor, and lift head up with a bounce three times.

2 Lift head and shoulders with a bounce.

3 Lift up from waist, bouncing three times.

4 Lift up from waist, with hands linked across chest, and bounce three times.

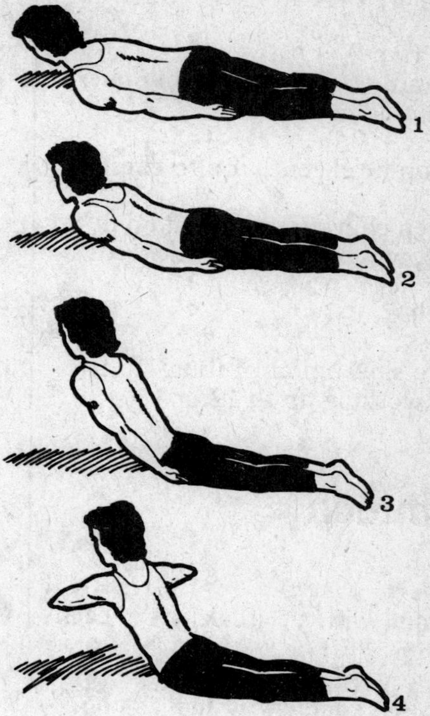

in chin

neck (*men*)

1 Stand, or sit, comfortably but keep shoulders well back.

2 Drop head gently on to chest.

3 Keep chin tucked in, and pull head slowly but firmly backwards.

4 Relax.

Hold to slow count of four. Do five times, working up to 12 or 15.

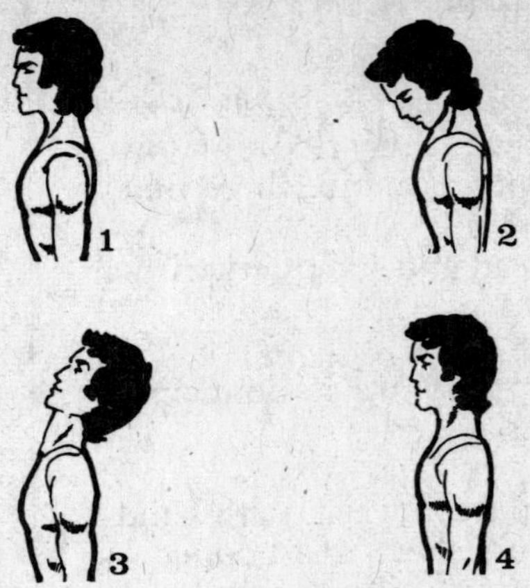

big hunch

shoulders (*men*)

1 Stand with a 5 lb weight in each hand.

2 Raise shoulders as high as you can.

3 Then press them hard together at back, so that shoulder blades are squeezed.

4 Drop shoulders.

5 Bring them hard forward and up.

6 Relax.

Do three times, increasing gradually to 10.

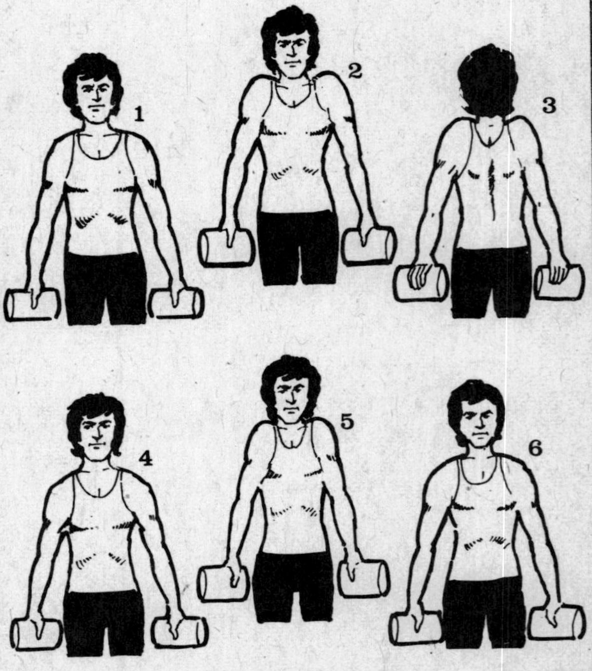

the one that got away

shoulders

1 Stand, feet slightly apart, arms at sides, gripping a 5 lb weight in each hand. Palms should face sides.

2 Slowly raise arms up and out to shoulder level.

3 Lower just as slowly.

Do three times, building up to 10.

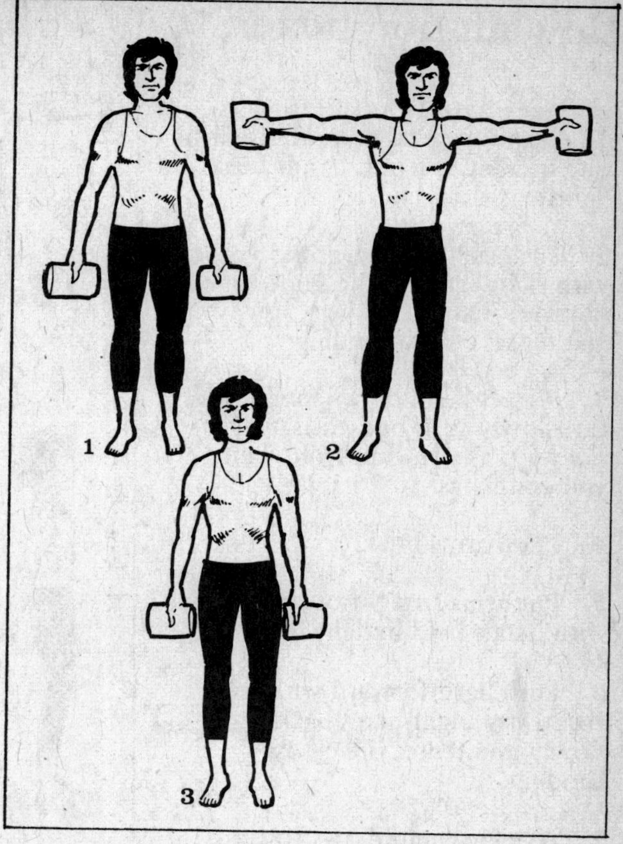

slow motion boxer

shoulders (*men*)
1 Stand, feet together, both arms out straight in front, hands held lightly as fists.

2 Push as hard forward as you can with right arm. At the same time, draw left hand back very slowly and tense, elbow bending.

3 As left hand draws towards left ear, slowly turn body as far left sideways as you can. Hold while you count fast to 20.

4 Drop arms briskly.

5 Put arms straight out in front, with hands held in light fists.

6 Push hard forward with left arm. Draw right hand back very slowly and tense, the elbow bending.

7 As right hand draws towards right ear, slowly turn body as far right sideways as possible. Hold for a fast count of 20.

8 Drop arms briskly.

Do three times with each arm. Work up gradually to eight or 10 with right arm out, then with the left arm. Breathe evenly throughout.

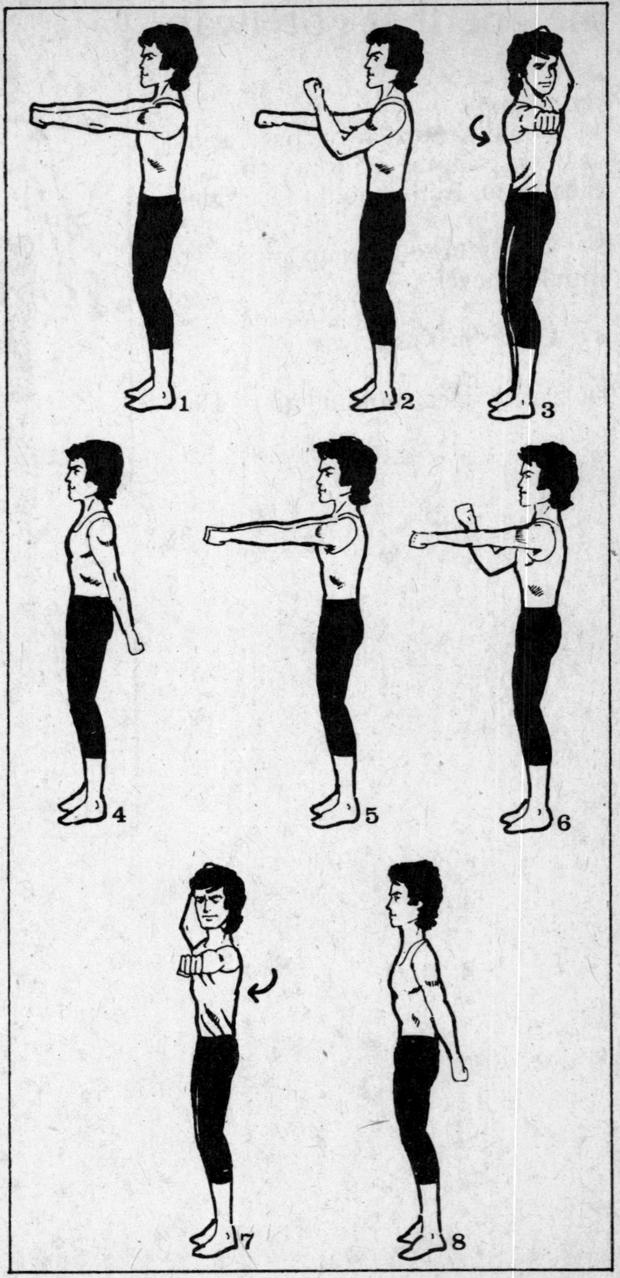

two up, two down

shoulders and arms (*men*)
1 Stand, feet slightly apart, arms at sides, with 5 lb weight in each hand.

2 Slowly raise arms up and out straight at shoulder level.

3 Then up above the head.

4 Lower to shoulder level.

5 Then down to sides again.

Count one-two-three-four. Do exercise three times, working up to 10.

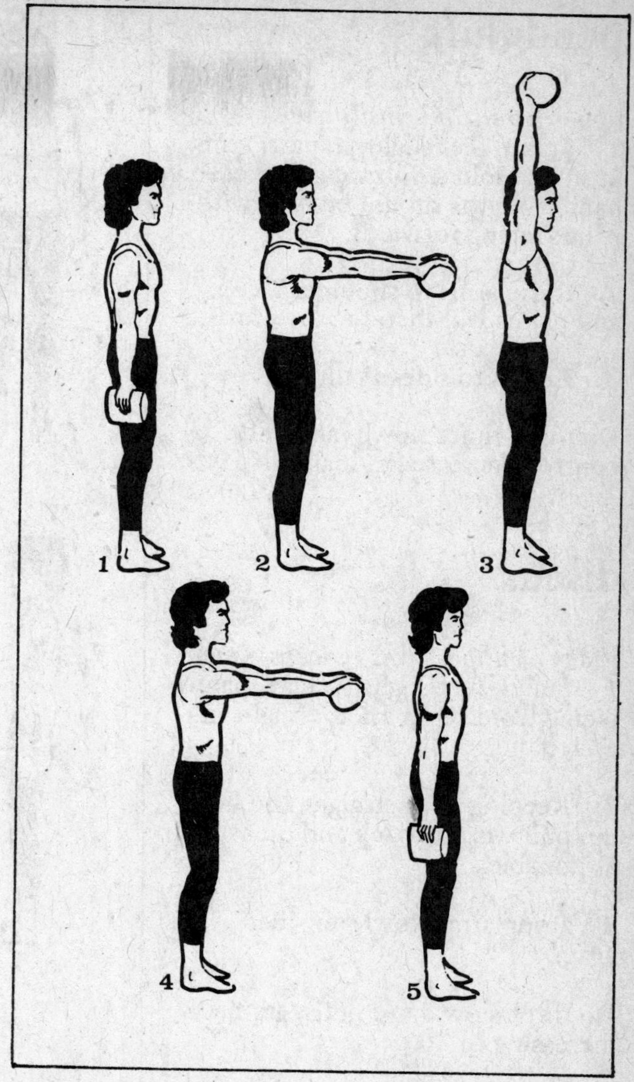

pendulum

upper fronts of arms (biceps)
1 Stand, feet slightly apart, arms at sides. Hold a 5 lb weight in each hand. Weights should be held with palms facing forwards.

2 Raise arms to shoulder level, and palms will then face upwards.

3 Lower to sides again.

Do three times slowly and with control. Increase gradually to 10.

discus

backs of upper arms (triceps) (men)
1 Stand, feet slightly apart, palms facing front. Grip a 5 lb weight in each hand.

2 Keeping back straight and head up, pull weights back and up as far as possible.

3 Bring arms slowly to sides again.

Do three slow, hard pulls, gradually increasing to 10.

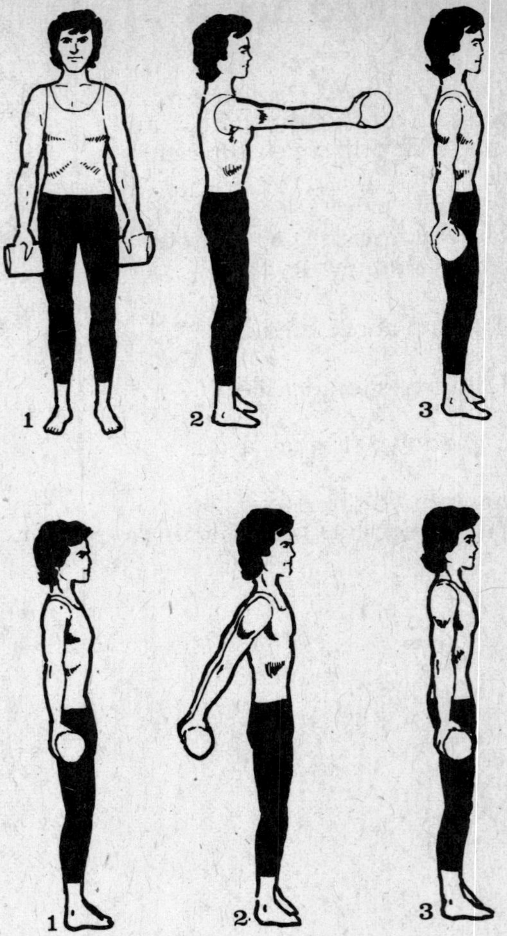

making the wheels go round

arms, mainly shoulders and elbows

1 Stand, with feet slightly apart, elbows bent, and a 5 lb weight held under chin with both hands.

2 Slowly press arms up to ceiling . . .

3 . . . then down forwards to rest in front of you.

Do three times, working up to 10.

(It's a good idea to practise this in conjunction with 'two up, two down', as each exercise works different sets of muscles.)

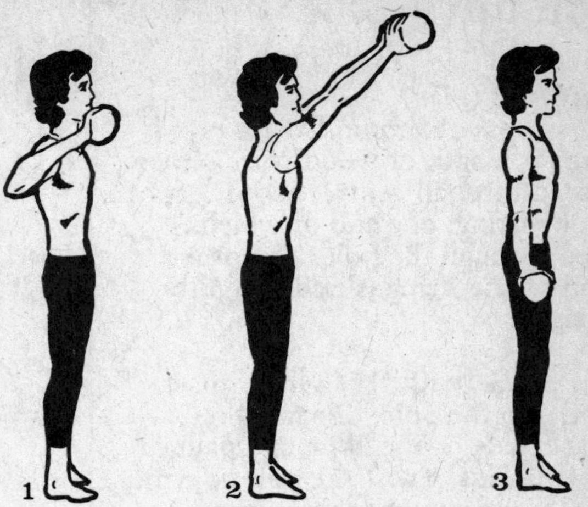

palm rolls

forearms

1 Lean arm firmly on the table and keep it there. Pluck up the end of a newspaper or cloth. Roll it into the palm and squeeze it hard into a ball. Do this five times with each hand. Build up to 10 times with each hand.

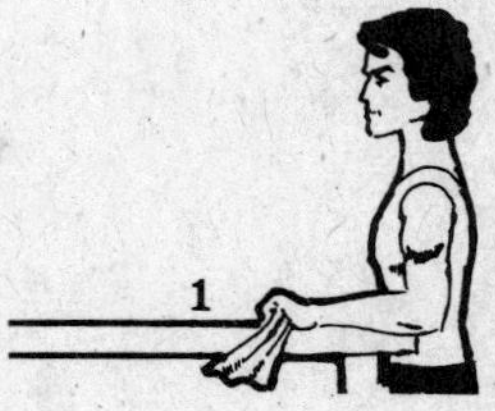

roll up

forearms (*men*)
You need: A broom handle or similar length of wood with a hole bored through centre, about 3 ft of stout string, one end of which is tied through the hole. The other end of the string is tied to a 5 lb weight.

1 Stand, with feet a little apart, and grip the pole, one hand on either side of the hole, and palms *downwards.* Twist the pole to wind up the string until the weight reached the pole. Do this three times.

2 Then do it three more times, but this time grip the broom with the palms *upwards*.

Work gradually up to 10 times (palms down, palms up).

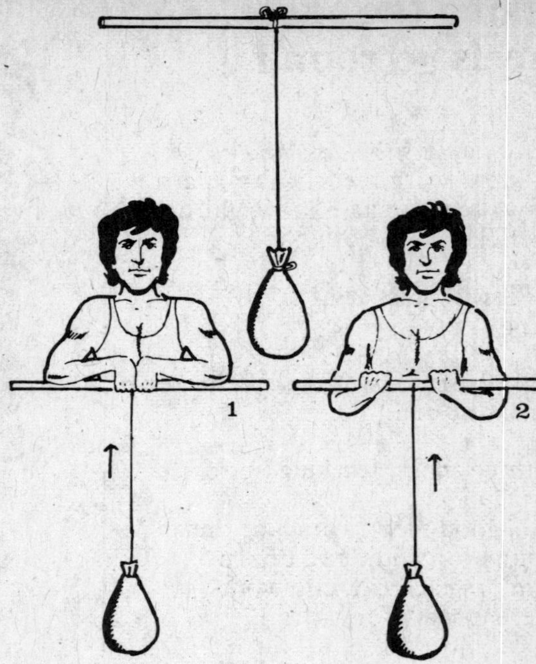

get to grips

hands (*isometric*)
1 and 2 Squeeze a squashy ball, having one in each hand or switching a ball from hand to hand. Do it when standing, sitting, anytime, anywhere. Any number of times.

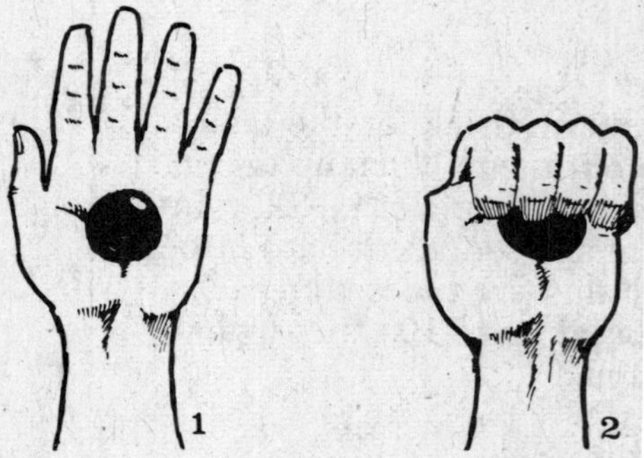

long reach

fighting a 'spare tyre'
1 and 2 Lie down, with knees bent up.

3 Reach with right arm down right side, as far as you can, without raising trunk.

4 Go back to first position.

5 Then reach with left arm down left side, as far as you can, without raising trunk.

6 Return to first position.

Count one-two-three-four. Do three times, working up to 10.

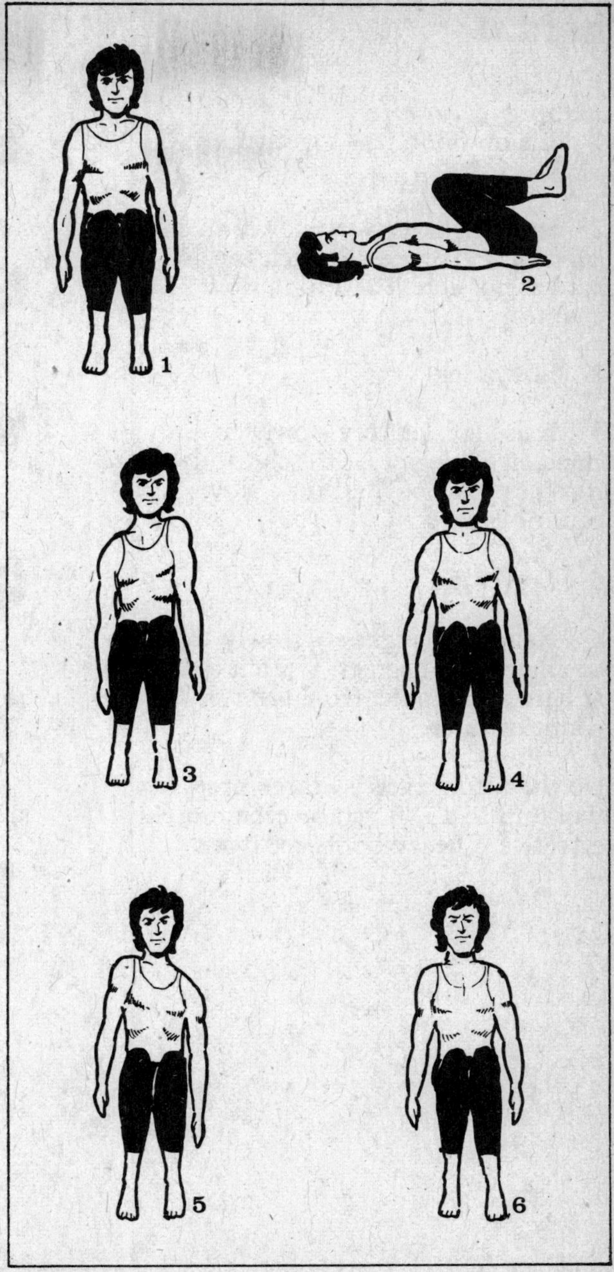

hold it

abdomen easier
1 Lie on floor, legs together, arms at sides.

2 Raise right leg very slowly to an angle of 45 degrees. Stretch toe as hard as possible. Hold for a slow count of three.

3 Lower leg.

4 Raise left leg very slowly to an angle of 45 degrees. Stretch toe as hard as possible. Hold for a slow count of three.

5 Lower leg.

6 Raise both legs very slowly to an angle of 45degrees. Stretch toes as hard as possible. Hold for a slow count of three.

Do the whole exercise three times. Work up to 15. It can be even more effective if heavy boots are worn.

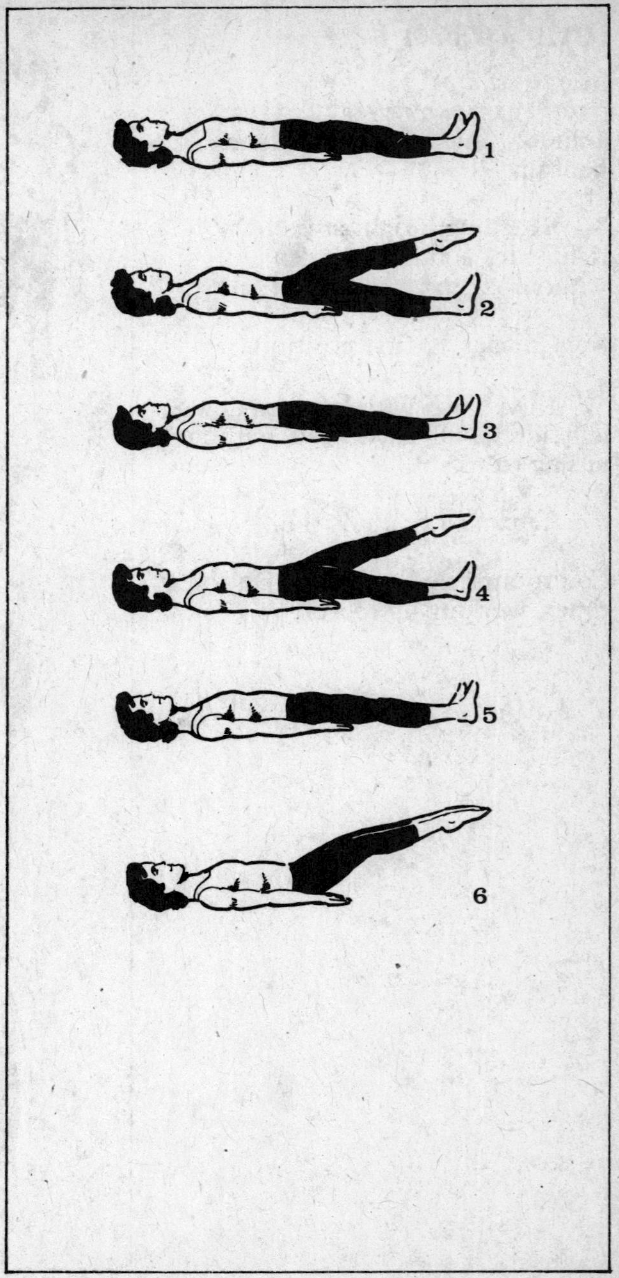

Australian cyclist

abdomen (*with bonus of leg toning*)
1 Lie on back, on floor, with arms straight at sides.

2 Raise trunk off floor, legs straight up in air. Take weight on arms and hands to lever you up. Bend elbows and place hands behind hip bones to support, so only shoulders are on floor. Start cycling in air. Keep legs circling as high and wide as you can. Try to push toes ever further up at highest point of each revolution. 10 revolutions each leg to begin. Gradually add more and cycle faster – still keeping circles wide.

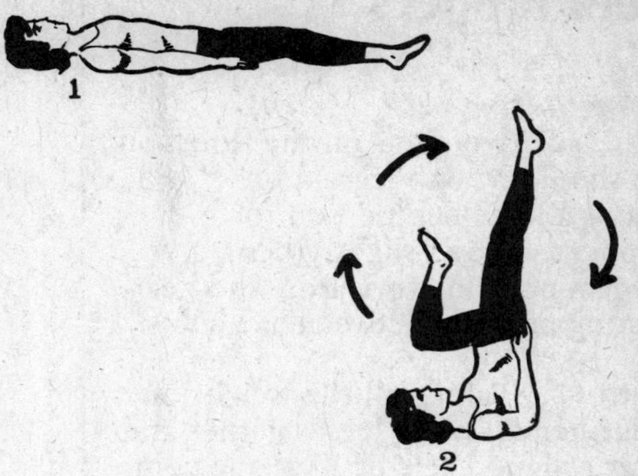

look no hammock

abdomen (*men*)
1 Sit, with legs out straight and tilted upwards, by resting feet on a low stool, a chair, or against wall. Grip hands behind head.

2 Round the upper part of the body and 'sink' heavily against the hands, rather as if in a hammock. You should feel the pull in the abdomen and diaphragm. Slowly curl head into knees.

3 Uncurl back to rounded position.

Do exercise three times, gradually working up to 10. The higher the legs go, the more effective the exercise.

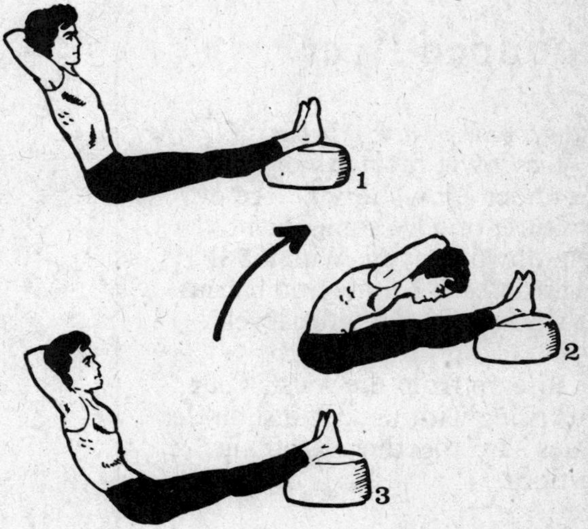

heel tappers

strengthening back (*men*)

1 Place two coins on the floor. Sit on the floor with legs straight, and hands a little behind you for support, elbows slightly bent, fingers pointing forwards, and heels resting midway between the coins.

2 to 4 Taking all the weight on your hands, swing legs together and over to land heels first by one coin, then by the other.

Do 15 times on each side quickly, increasing to 30 times on each side.

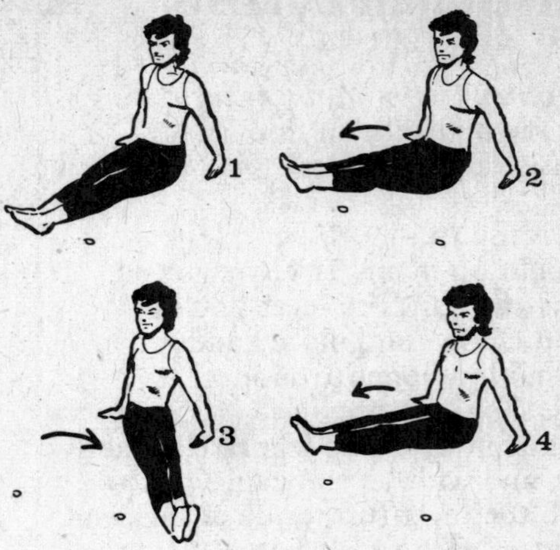

grounded flyer

strengthening back (*men*)

1 Lie down, facing floor, with feet under a low, heavy piece of furniture, or have someone hold them down for you. With a 5 lb weight in each hand, stretch arms out sideways at shoulder level.

2 Rise up from the waist, your arms rising with you. Pull shoulder blades hard together. Keep hips on the floor.

3 Lower.

Do exercise three times rhythmically, up to a maximum of 10.

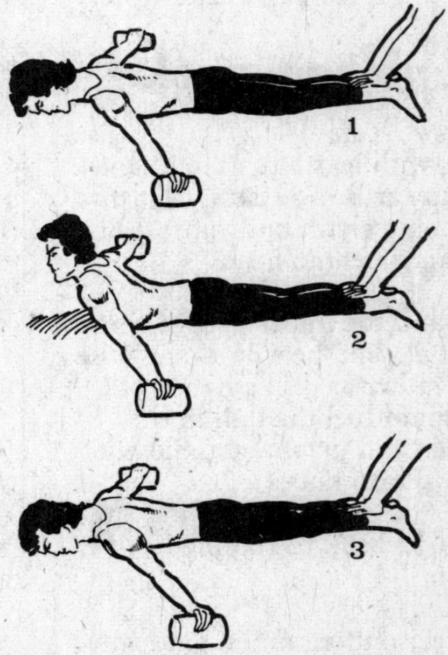

concertina

legs, especially thighs (*men*)

1 Stand, feet slightly apart, hands on hips.

2 Rise up on toes.

3 Bend knees and crouch down, sitting on heels.

4 Rise on to toes again.

5 Lower down on to heels.

Keep back straight throughout. Do exercise five times, working up to 15, and getting gradually faster.

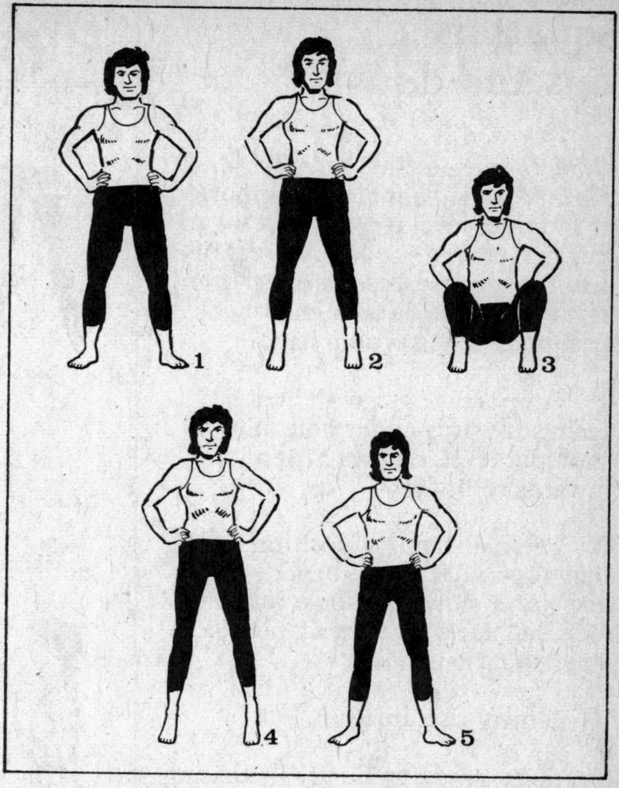

squatters
ups and downs

strengthening legs, especially knees
A 10 lb weight should be supported at shoulder level to give impetus to this movement – two 5 lb bags of potatoes, sawdust, sand or earth in stout bags, one at each end of a firm pole, like a broom handle.

1 Support weight with hands facing upwards under pole at shoulder level, elbows bent and inwards to body.

2 From a standing position, with feet about 1 ft apart, bend knees and lower slowly to squat halfway. You can use a stool as a guide to your squat position.

3 Slowly rise up again.

Do three times, gradually increasing to 10.

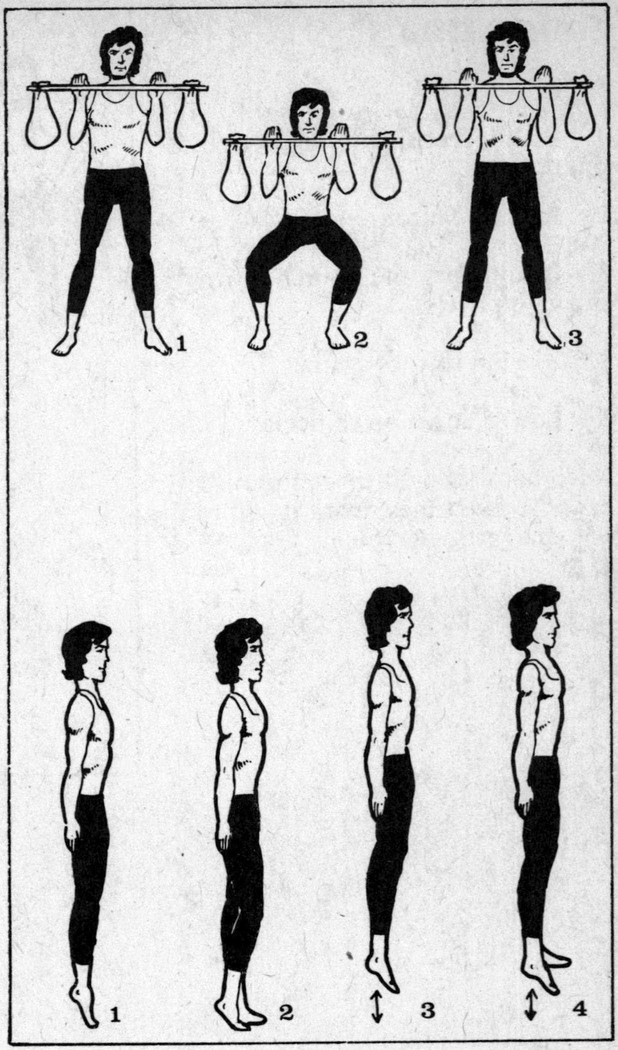

strong stand

calves
1 Standing, feet together, rise up on toes as high as you can go and lower again.

2 Rise on toes again but this time first on right leg then on left – five times.

3 Get on toes, jump off ground and land back on toes (can bend knees a little to lift you up) – five times.

4 Rising on toes of one leg, hop up and back on to toes. Then with the other leg. Five times each.

tailored tail

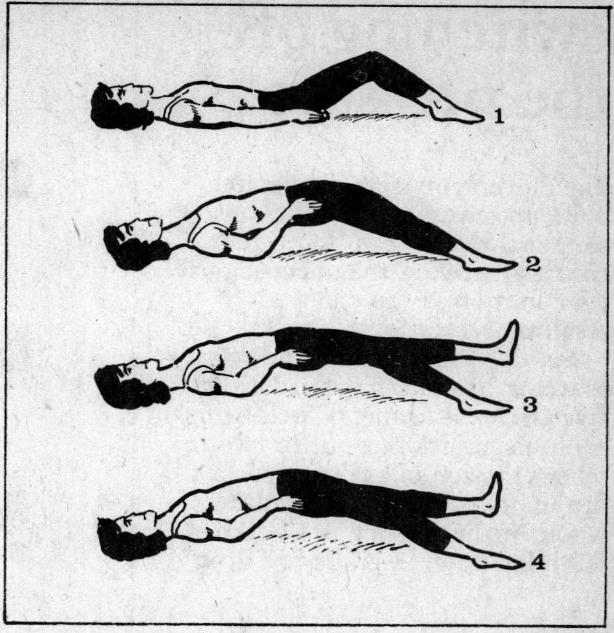

seat (*men*)

1 Lie on back with knees bent up, feet on ground.

2 Raise hips off ground as high as you can go. You're supported by shoulders and toes. Back to starting position.

3 Repeat stage 2 but lift right leg. Back to start.

4 Repeat exercise, but this time lift left leg instead of right. Back to starting position.

Toughish. Do exercise three times at first, working gradually up to 10.

switching off the pressure

The movements here deliberately build up tension within the muscles so that the body can 'learn' the contrast between the unconscious tension it builds up and the resultant relaxation.

So, they both pep up and relax, as well as stimulating circulation to give a general feeling of well-being.

You can pick out one or two to relieve tension in a particular part of the body, or run through the whole of them. They're all carried out lying down – on bed or floor.

(*men*)

1 Turn toes in towards you, bending foot from ankle.

2 Press backs of knees into bed or floor.

3 Press knees together.

4 Contract buttock muscles.

5 Place hand under small of back. Press down hard with back as if crushing hand.

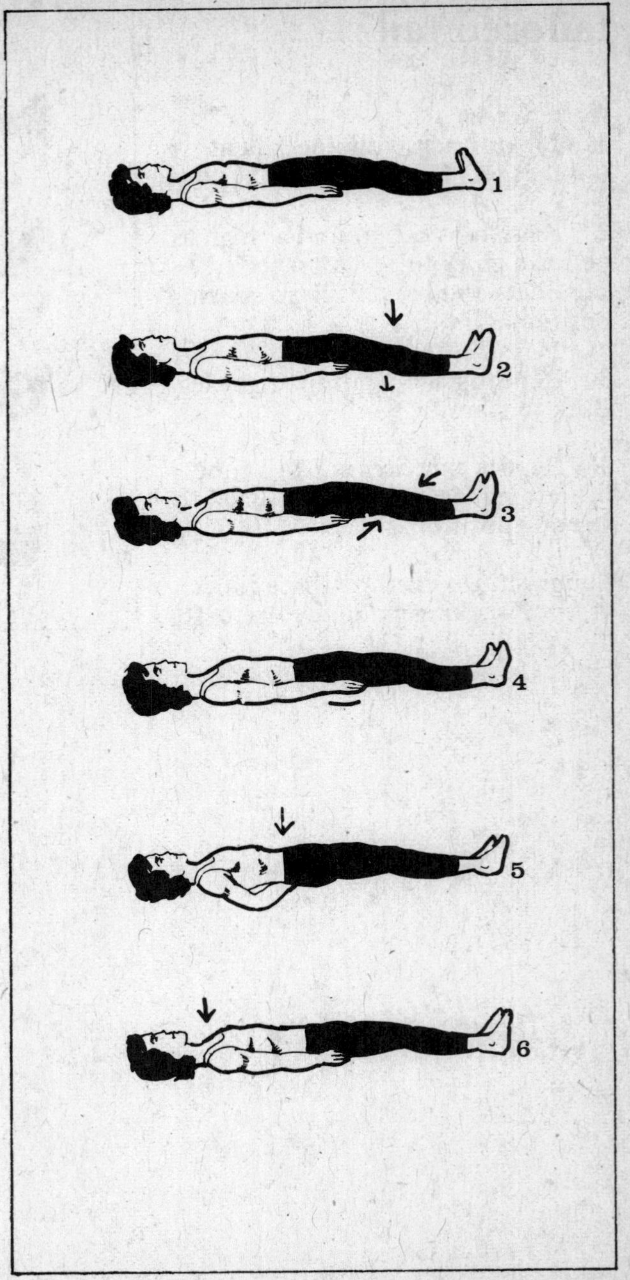

6 Arms at sides, press shoulders and elbows back into floor.

7 and 8 Clench and unclench fists in air.

9 and 10 Let hands flop on to stomach, then at sides.

11 Press head back hard into pillow or floor – feel neck muscles tighten.

As with business man's keep fit format: clench face muscles, squeeze up eyes, bare teeth, 'concertina' eyes. Pull as many facial expressions as you can manage.

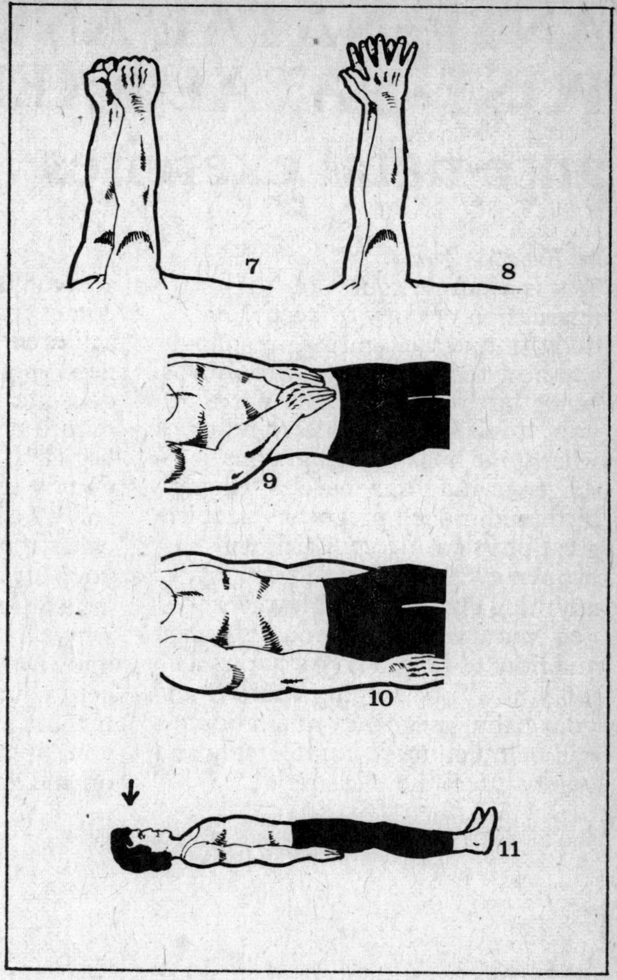

ANTE-NATAL AND POST-NATAL EXERCISES

ante-natal exercises

by Erna Wright

This is a simple course of instruction on how to keep your body fit and well during pregnancy and how to prepare your 'tools' for giving birth to your baby. What are your 'tools'? Your understanding of what your body is doing, your diligence and your muscles. Giving birth and indeed pregnancy require great physical effort which will happen even if you don't do anything consciously. However if you know what your body is doing and how to help it to carry out its job you will be helping yourself and your baby, pregnancy and labour will be much more comfortable and you will feel the pleasure of accomplishment which always comes from something one has achieved by one's own efforts. You need to practise regularly and that does mean every day after the 4th month of pregnancy until labour begins. Get your husband to help you by supervising your daily 'stint' and by checking that you are doing 'what the book says', exactly. If your local hospital offers classes in 'relaxation', attend them – they won't hurt. But tell the doctor and midwife that you are preparing to help yourself during labour as well. If there are no classes available in your area – don't despair, just read on and go to it!

new muscles at work

When you begin to learn and practise the exercises in this section, you should realise that each exercise has a special purpose, which is explained. Don't rush in after a tiring day and flop down and hurry through your exercises as if you were putting your make-up on. Your nervous system can't develop skills unless you allot a special unrushed period of time each day. If you occasionally have a particularly harrassed day, leave the practising until order has been restored the next day. (Don't make this excuse to yourself too often!)

Your exercises should be done on the floor rather than on your bed — a bed is usually too comfortable and you can't feel the exact sensations in your muscles too well if your mattress hugs you too cosily. Collect as many cushions and pillows as you need on the floor to make yourself comfortable there. (A thin foam mattress like the ones sold for sun-bathing on the beach, is excellent as a base, plus the cushions.)

1 This is your basic position; but vary the number of pillows under your head and shoulders to your own needs.

2 The wedge shape under the knees (very necessary for correct support during exercises and during early labour) can be made from foam rubber stitched into a piece of washable material. The thin end points towards your seat.

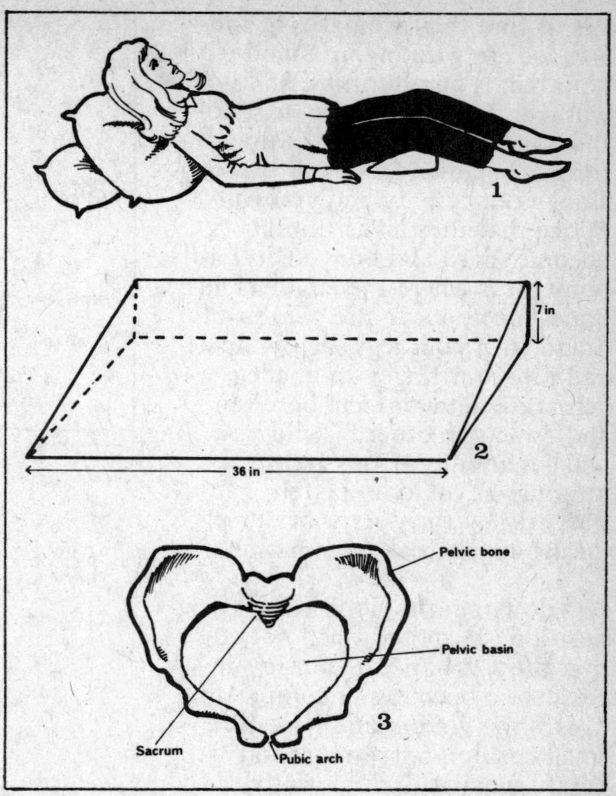

3 Let us find out what the muscles which you must learn to use are doing and how to use them. The *pelvis*, shown here, consists of two identical bones at the sides joined by a triangular bone at the back called the *sacrum.* The pelvic bones meet in front to form the *pubic arch.*

Continued overleaf

Let us find the landmarks of the area we are working in. Stand with your hands on your hips, and you will feel the upper outer ridges of the bones of your pelvis. Run your forefinger down from your navel along your tummy and you will notice that the elastic tummy becomes hard and bony. This hard bony bit is where the large pelvic bones meet, above the *pubic arch*. Stand with your legs slightly apart and run your finger up one leg, across the bony area in between and down the other leg and you will get an idea of this arch although it can only be felt properly by the doctor or nurse during an internal examination.

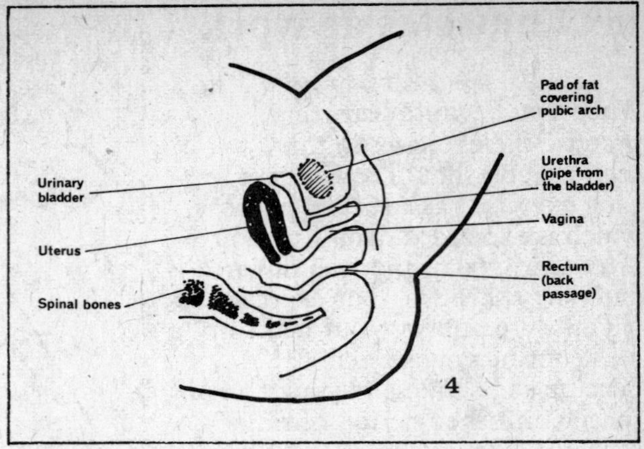

Lay down on the floor in the basic position (1) and you will notice that the flat bone in your lower back soon becomes uncomfortable. This is the *sacrum* and it needs a small cushion for support and comfort particularly during pregnancy when the shape of your body is constantly changing. Hanging from the sacrum is a little tail of five small bones all fused together, the *coccyx*. All these bones and associated muscles are known together as the *pelvic basin*.

4 In both men and women the organs of reproduction are housed in this basin. The shape of the male pelvic basin is much narrower and more triangular than the female one. In the middle of the female pelvic basin we find the *womb* or *uterus* – both being official words for the organ which is the baby's nursery until he is developed enough to live outside your body. The uterus is about the size of a pear when a woman is not pregnant but by the time she is 12 weeks pregnant it begins to overspill into the tummy because it is too big for the pelvic basin. The uterus goes on growing as the baby grows and it is this growth which gives a pregnant woman her special shape.

5 The pelvic basin has a bottom of flesh or muscles called the *pelvic floor.* The pelvic floor will come into action during the actual birth of your baby and therefore we must make sure that all the muscles of the pelvic floor are supple and elastic. So several exercises will be designed for that purpose.

When you exercise the muscles must work harder and use more body-fuel. To do this efficiently they need oxygen, so always do your exercises in a *room with an open window.*

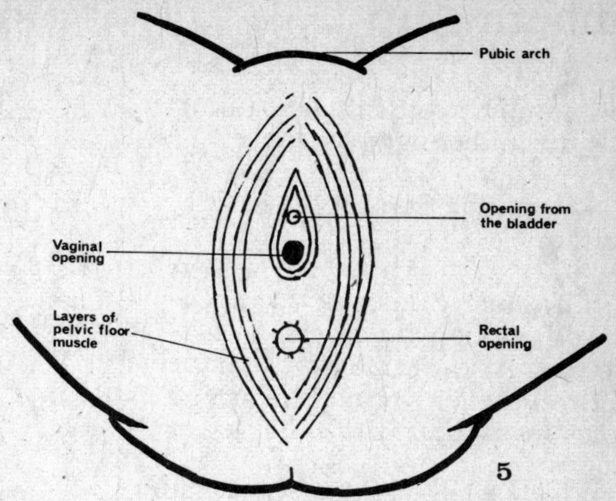

5

conscious controlled breathing

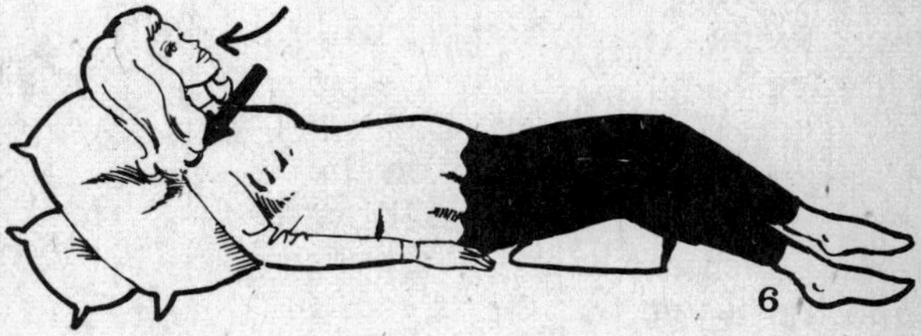

6

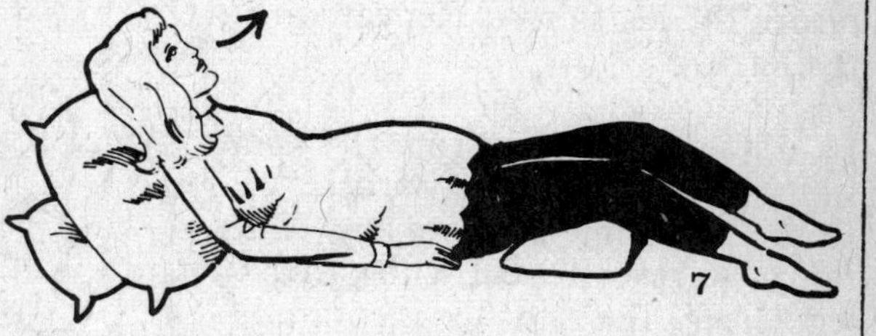

7

Every athlete learns this and, in a way, having a baby is an athletic performance. A word of warning! Giving the body too much oxygen by breathing too fast or too strenuously is also not good, so please be exact and keep your conscious breathing steady and regular. You will need several different levels of conscious breathing during labour, but the first set of exercises go with *Level A* breathing which is as follows:

1 Breathe in through the nose with the mouth closed, using chest muscles. Push shoulders back when breathing in.

2 Blow out through mouth, as though blowing on soup. Notice how the chest sags.

Practise the breathing for about half a minute and try to get four to six breaths in and out during that time. If you feel slightly dizzy afterwards, make your effort more gentle and take it more slowly – three to four breaths in half a minute. Keep the rhythm steady.

limbering up

Now combine conscious breathing with the limbering-up exercises.

1 Lay on the floor in the basic position.

2 Lift one leg, keeping the knee straight, as high as you can with comfort. At the same time breathe in. Drop the leg down again as you blow out. Repeat with other leg.

3 Lift left leg slightly and swing it out sideways, without tilting your hips. Swing it back. Repeat with right leg.

4 Grasp the right ankle on the inside with the right hand. Breathe in and push the knee towards the floor until you feel the stretch in the inner thigh. Blow out as you return the leg to rest. Repeat with the left leg.

5 Lift the right leg from the knee support and turn it outwards. Rotate the foot six times and return to rest. Repeat with other leg. (*Note:* the right leg is rotated clockwise, and the left leg anti-clockwise.) Each of the limbering-up exercises should be done once a day. Take care to time the beginning of each exercise with the beginning of the controlled breath as this gives you good practice for what you will do later during labour rehearsals and during labour itself.

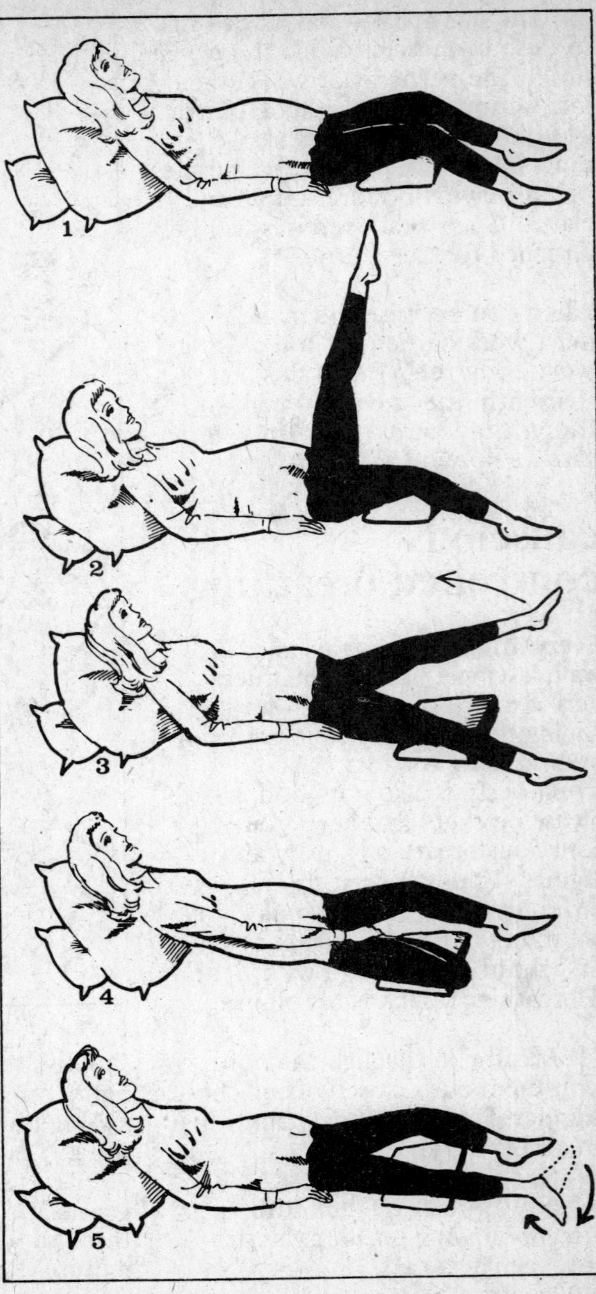

muscle contraction and decontraction

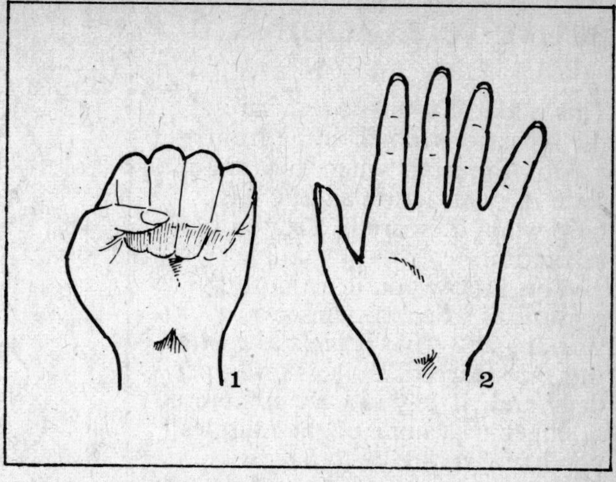

1 and 2 When a group of muscles performs its action its threads or fibres shorten and thicken. (Make a fist with the muscles of your hand and you will see this clearly.) This shortening/thickening action is called a *contraction.*

The uterus or womb is a muscle-bag, so it works by contracting also. The important difference between the muscles of the uterus and the muscles of the hand is that we contract the hand muscles by an act of will, while the uterus is controlled by hormones and works independently of conscious control. During labour the uterus contracts at intervals so that the baby is pushed out through the narrow end of the uterus into the birth-canal and so is finally born. After each contraction of a group of muscles, the fibres lengthen and become thinner again and we call this the decontraction of muscles, which results in *relaxation.*

active relaxation

This is a drill to make us aware of the sensations which come from a group of muscles when they are in a state of contraction and how it feels when they are in a state of relaxation.

This is how you learn both the sensations when muscles are working and what it feels like when they are relaxed. Do this drill once daily and, after you have completed it, check that none of the muscles you have worked with have inadvertently contracted while you were doing something else. If they have, correct them.

1 and 2 Contract the right leg, then the left leg. The pelvic muscles should then be contracted, then the chest and shoulder muscles, and finally the face muscles.

At the end of the whole drill you will be in a lovely relaxed state but there is no point in staying that way. During labour this state will only last a short time in between the powerful contractions of the uterus, so now prepare the body to become active once more. The whole action-rate of the body has been slowed down by this exercise and must be increased *gradually*. Never jump up suddenly after this exercise – you may feel giddy or faint.

3 and 4 Clench and unclench the hands, and at the same time wiggle the feet. Then get up slowly.

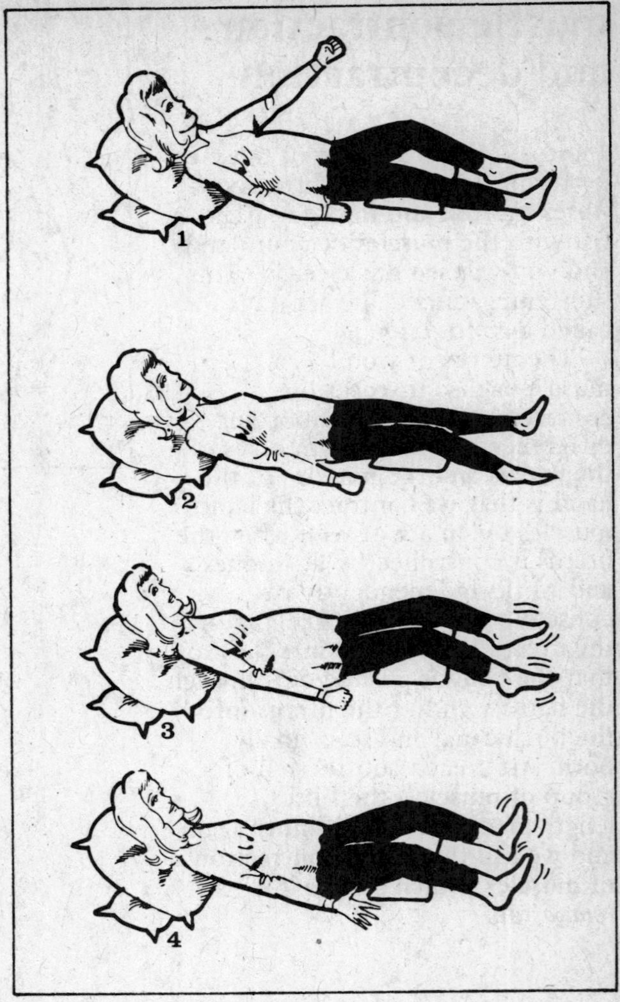

getting up

Usually after lying down we raise our bodies by using our tummy-muscles. This is too strenuous during pregnancy. This applies to getting up after doing your exercises, getting up from the bath and getting out of bed.

1 to 4 This shows the correct way to get up. Do as slowly as you can – think of a slow motion film and you'll get the idea.

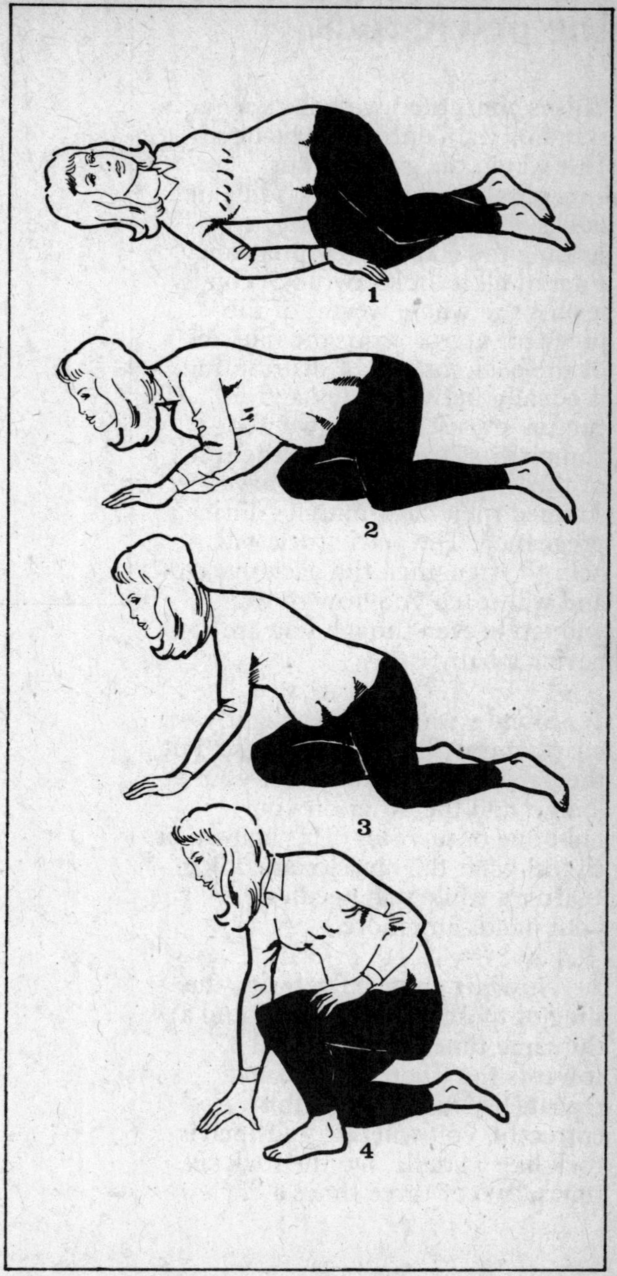

the pelvic rock

This is concerned with the way you stand or walk during pregnancy. Just watch the girls in your ante-natal clinic – they waddle like ducks, especially those who are nearing the end of their pregnancy. First of all it looks awful. Secondly, it puts the whole weight of the pregnant uterus on to the muscles of the back instead of distributing it equally between back and tummy-muscles. Many women complain of backache for the rest of their lives because they have strained their back-muscles during pregnancy. The pelvic rock will help to strengthen the back-muscles and will teach you how to walk with style even though you are having a baby.

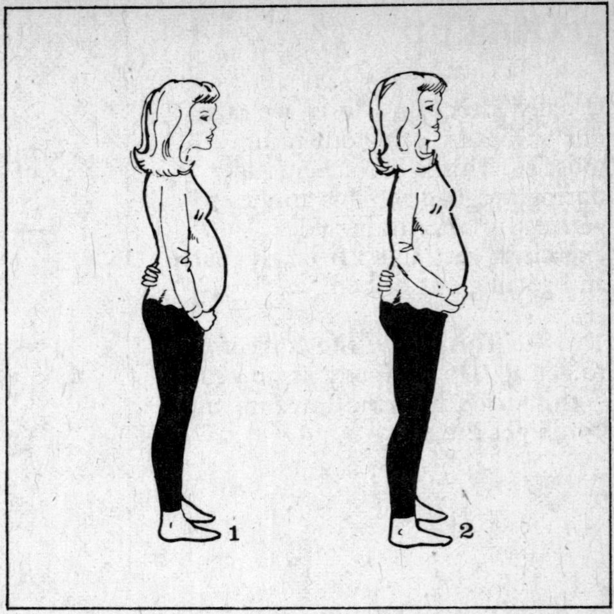

1 Stand with your feet slightly apart, and with the knees loose. Put the palm of one hand under your 'bulge' and the other on your tail-bone or *sacrum.* (This helps you to feel what the muscles are doing – after a while you needn't use your hands any more.)

2 Now lift your 'bulge' with the sling of muscles underneath, and at the same time push your tail towards the floor. Release and repeat. If you are doing this correctly, you will feel your pelvis rock like a cradle. Do the rock six times, two or three times a day.

3 and 4 In addition, whenever you are walking or standing, particularly when you are carrying a shopping-bag, do the first half of the exercise. Notice how much nicer figure 4 looks and how much better the clothes hang. Don't forget to keep your shoulders back – the exercise is impossible to do properly with rounded shoulders.

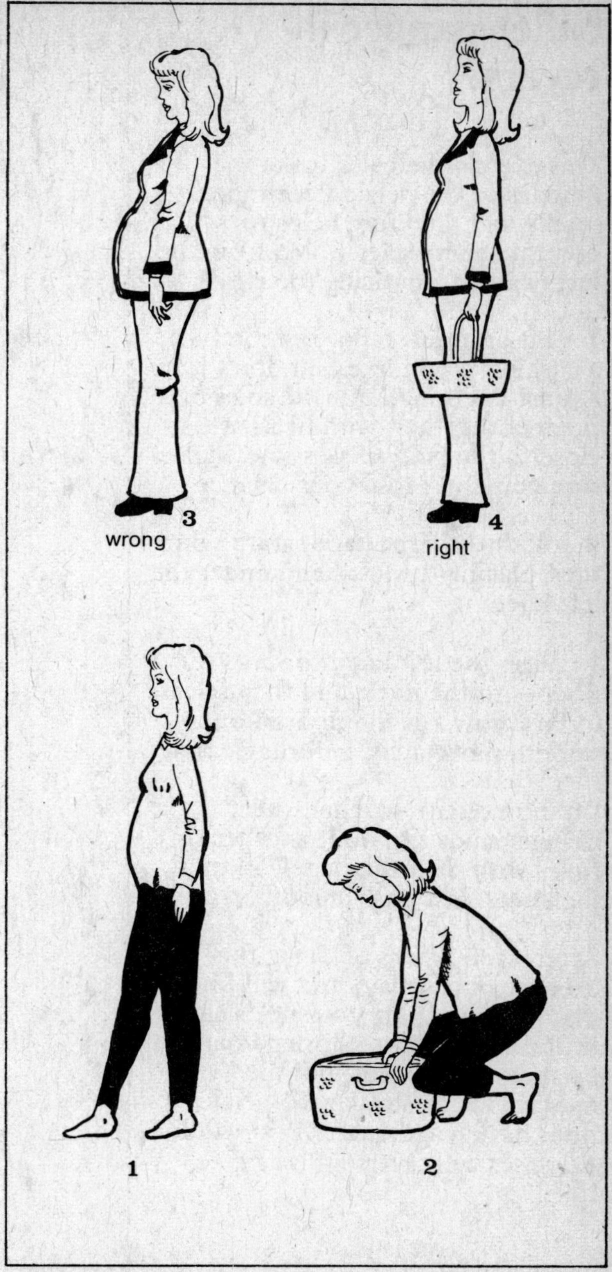

lifting

How to lift anything at any time, is a piece of very practical know-how for you, your husband or anyone else who must inevitably bend down to pick up something they have dropped or a heavy object.

1 Stand with one foot in front of the other.

2 Bend both knees as you move towards the ground. When you start lifting, make the thigh muscles, rather than the tummy muscles, take the load.

ballet-dancer in reverse

This exercise helps to make the muscles of the pelvic floor more supple and therefore helps to prevent the muscles which form the birth-canal from being too rigid.

1 Sit on floor, tailor-fashion (use a cushion if you like, but don't lean against anything). Put the soles of the feet together, with heels as close to the body as possible. Make sure you don't lose your balance.

2 With the right hand, grasp your toes, placing the left hand under the left knee.

3 Push the left hand towards the floor with the knee, and then release it. Push towards the floor in one smooth movement, before releasing.

Do the exercise six times, then change hands and do it another six times with the other leg. Don't jerk the knees, just push smoothly.

After a few weeks of doing this exercise once a day, you will find that you can bring your heels closer to the body without losing your balance – the proof that the muscles which stretch the pelvic floor have lengthened. (Post-natal exercises will reverse this again.)

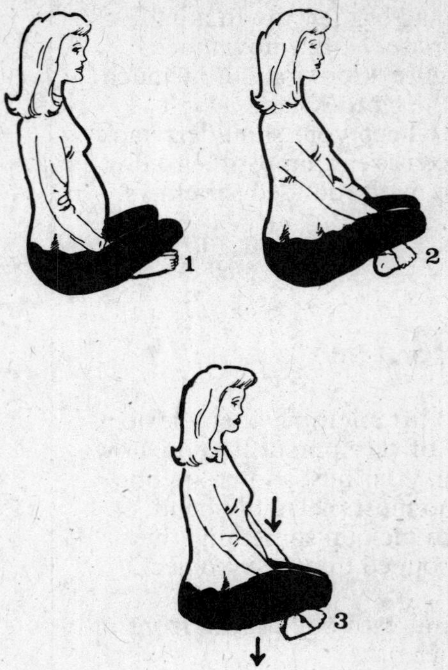

muscles covering the back of pelvis

The best treatment for chronic backache. Practise it now and use it, if you need to. It is very helpful in early labour if backache is experienced. (In labour it should be done together with the appropriate breathing-technique.)

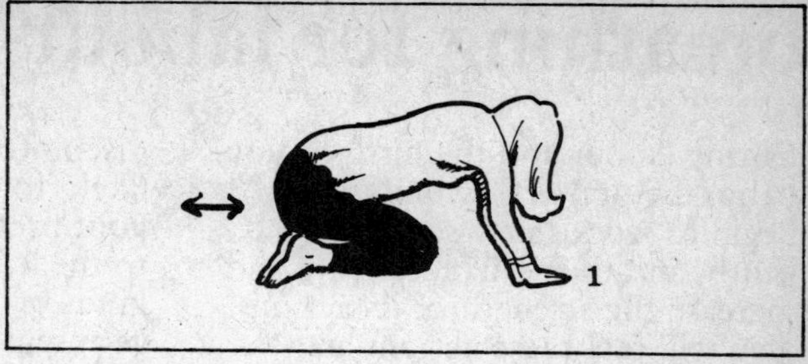

1 Kneel on the floor, sitting back on your heels. Rest your hands on the floor in front of you, with the elbows turned outwards and slightly bent. Put your head down and hump your back. Now, using your thigh-muscles like pistons, push your buttocks out backwards – like a duck lifting its tail. Feel your thigh-muscles doing the work. Then make them pull your buttocks back again, as though you were trying to hide them. Repeat six times.

square bears

This exercise is almost impossible to do correctly at first – persevere and it will come.

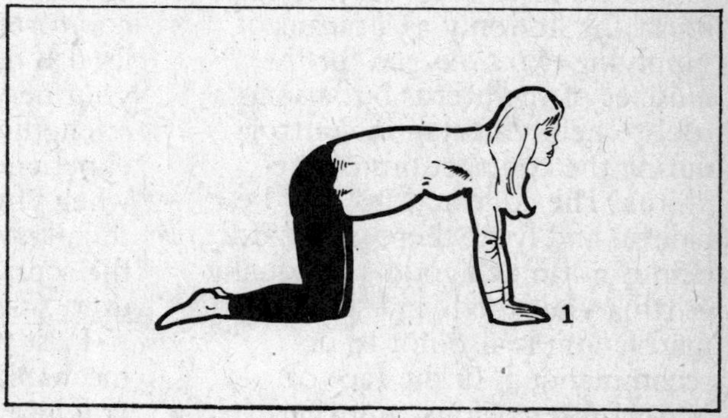

1 Kneel on the floor, with your knees slightly apart. Put your hands flat on the floor – arms straight. Your back should be arched slightly upwards, so that your body forms a square between knees and hands. (Like a bear standing still.)
Contract the muscles surrounding the *back passage* only, and release, then contract the muscles surrounding the *front passage* (these include those of the vagina or *birth canal* and of the bladder) and release. Lastly contract all the muscles of the *pelvic floor* and release.

Do this pattern three times, once a day. At first you will almost certainly not be able to isolate the different groups nor will you feel that you have, with certainty. After a few weeks, if you keep on trying, you will succeed, and this control will help you enormously during the actual birth of the baby.

breathing for labour

During labour and the birth of your baby, the uterus or womb will begin to work fairly slowly and gently and then will accelerate and increase the strength of its actions. You will feel these actions as wave-like, tightening around your tummy and perhaps your back – in other words all around 'your bulge'. You will also feel the relaxation of the muscles which follows.

You would find, if you tried it, that if you used level A breathing only, supposing you knew no other, it would not be a good enough help when the muscles of the womb really get going with their work. Try to think of your controlled breathing not only as a means of supplying extra oxygen for the muscles of the uterus but also as a tool to help you stay in control during the contractions of the uterus. The contractions may be painful and lying there yelling for help is not much good and equally gritting your teeth and suffering martyrdom is also not to be recommended. In the face of powerful sensations, anywhere in the body, the correct response is one which is equally powerful without using unduly muscles other than those being used for the job in hand.

This sounds very scientific and complicated but I'll give you something to practise on, which will prove that *you can* use conscious control when meeting discomfort. I am sure that you are likely to go to the dentist's during your pregnancy or even more likely to the hairdressers. I dislike both kinds of 'treatment'. My gums are very sensitive to touch and my scalp is equally so.

When the dentist probes or the hairdresser gives your head a good rub or when she pulls with brush or comb, just run over your muscles and deliberately decontract them – like a pilot doing a flight-deck check before take-off. Then start your controlled breathing in response to the sensations you feel – perhaps level A breathing is enough to help you feel moderately comfortable, but you might need level B or even C. That depends on your nervous system and the strength of pull or pressure you experience. But you will know when you are 'on top' and you will then know what you must do when the sensations come from the uterus during labour.

First we learn the breathing as a mechanical exercise, and then when you have become good at it, we shall learn to combine it with practice-labour exercises. Don't begin this until you are about six months pregnant.

Sit upright on a chair, and spread your palms at the bottom of your ribcage, just above your bulge. Have the fingertips meet. Now, with your mouth closed, take a deep breath, expanding your chest; then blow the air out through your mouth, just as you did in *conscious controlled breathing, A.*

After two or three breaths like this, move your hands up so that you feel your ribs moving and, with your mouth slightly open, breathe in and out, a little less deeply than before. Notice that now your ribs are expanding and relaxing as you breathe – this is *controlled breathing, B.*

Now after a few breaths in level B move your hands up to rest on your breast-bone and breathe still more lightly than before. Feel the breast-bone going in and out. Think of the word 'out' as you breathe out each time. The in breath follows naturally – this is *controlled breathing, C.*

Now relax your chest and shoulders completely and don't concentrate on your breathing any longer; just let it happen naturally. Instead think of a song which you like and whose words you know. Use a pop song or a ballad with a good rollicking rhythm. Instead of controlling your breathing, sing the song in your head, mime the words with your lips and tap the rhythm with your fingers in your lap. Always use the same song when you practise and in labour also – make it Your Song.

Exaggerate the miming with your lips, because this helps your muscle-control in labour as you will find – this is *controlled breathing D.*

Practise this breathing exercise each day, using about half a minute for each level; try to make the change-over from one level to another smooth and change immediately without having to think. If you are a car driver, think of this as learning to change gear and you will know exactly what is meant.

the secret weapon

By now you are doing your ante-natal keep-fit every day and you are just going into your seventh month of pregnancy. You are skilled at using your conscious controlled breathing and your change-over from one level to another is smooth.

What now? How will all this help you during labour? Will you succeed or fail? Let's take the last question first – you can't fail. What is failure? You are not in a competition, you are trying to do what you can to help yourself during the birth of your baby. During those hours when your womb will slowly release the baby into your vagina or birth-canal, when the sensations become more and more powerful, you will do something to keep the feeling that you are not doing badly. You will be able to make use of drugs which help to relieve pain, if the doctor or midwife thinks you must have them, but your own control is valuable in addition, because it is you doing something for yourself and because you will not be exhausted by suffering needlessly.

Your whole body will be fresher and doing something in any situation is better than sitting or lying helplessly. You already know this from other crisis-situations you have handled. Labour is a peak-performance crisis situation for the body and particularly for the nervous system.

But in order to be able to help yourself, you must now practise the following exercises so regularly that doing what they teach you becomes an *automatic response.* How does it do that? If you teach your nervous system something, and practise it regularly at frequent intervals, it becomes automatic when you give the command.

labour drill – one

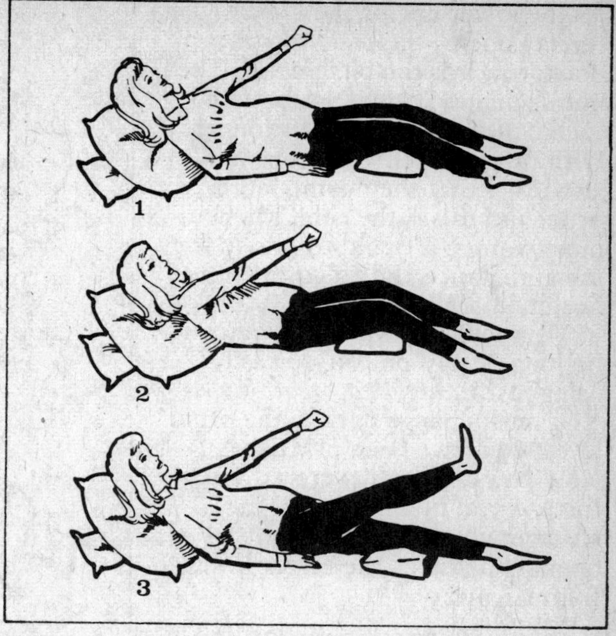

The purpose of this drill is to 'pretend' a contraction of the uterus during the early part of labour when the lower end of the womb begins to open and when the sensations are still fairly gentle. They will last about half to three quarters of a minute and this will be the time when you can still be at home doing light housework, but stopping to breathe your way through each contraction. Our pretend-uterus has to be a group of muscles which we can order to contract or decontract, but while using, say, your arm as your 'pretend' uterus, you must constantly check that no other muscles have joined in as well. The exercise is as follows:

1 Lay in the basic position. Use your left arm as the 'pretend' uterus and keep it tightly contracted, while breathing *controlled breathing A.* Check that all other muscles are relaxed. Keep this up for about 30 seconds, then slowly decontract while still doing the breathing until the arm is completely relaxed.

2 After doing this rest for a few minutes and then change over to using your right arm as your 'pretend' uterus. Repeat the breathing and checking other muscles as before. Keep going for 30 seconds, then relax for a few minutes.

3 Your 'pretend' uterus is now your right leg and left arm. Hold this contraction and Level A breathing for about 45–50 seconds then slowly decontract but maintain the breathing until all muscles are resting. Rest for a few minutes.

4 Now use your left leg and right arm as your 'pretend' uterus. Hold for 45–50 seconds then slowly decontract.

Continued overleaf

As the lower end of the *uterus* (the *cervix*) opens, the baby moves down towards the birth-canal. The uterus makes stronger efforts and each contraction also lasts longer. With the stronger sensations it is also usual that they come more often and this is the time when most women are told to phone for the ambulance and to go to hospital.

You will also find that you can no longer 'stay on top' so easily using just *Controlled breathing A*. You must change over to the other levels you have been practising. Now you can drop exercises 1 to 4. Instead you now 'pretend' the stronger contractions of the opening phase of the cervix in the following way:

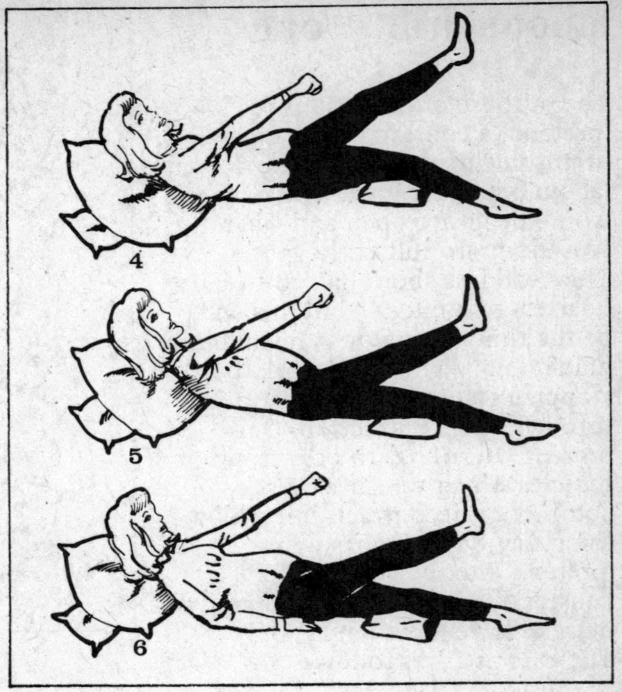

5 While doing a 'pretend' uterus contraction of the right arm/left leg, begin with *Controlled breathing A* for about 3 breaths then change to *Controlled breathing B* for about 5–6 breaths then to *Controlled breathing C* for about 8–10 breaths. For about 15–20 seconds sing your tune in your head and mime with your lips – tap the rhythm lightly with the fingers of the other hand. Finally come down through the levels of breathing again as you gradually decontract your 'pretend' uterus and do not forget to check all the time that no other muscles have joined in the contractions.

6 After a couple of minutes' rest, change your 'pretend' uterus to left arm/right leg and repeat the controlled breathing through all four levels up and down. It is easier to develop the skill of doing this if someone else helps you. They tell you when your 'pretend' contraction begins and when it gets 'pretend' stronger; in other words, when to change breathing levels. Your helper also tells you when it gets weaker and when it has gone.

In this way you learn to make immediate responses to signals, you are not consciously controlling – you don't control the sensations from your uterus in labour either. The more regular your practice is beforehand, the more will you be able to make the right responses during labour.

labour drill – two

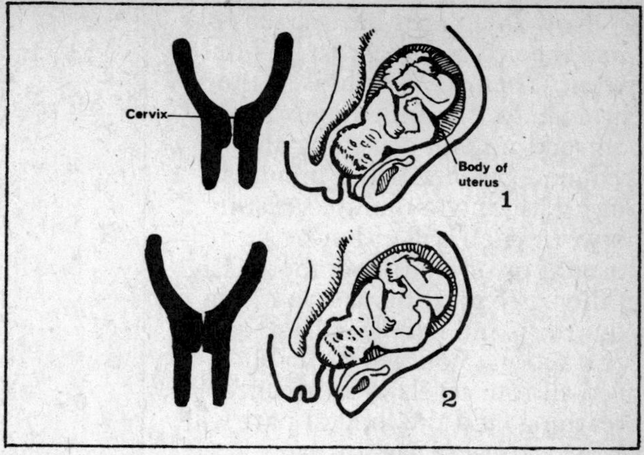

1 At the end of pregnancy, but before labour begins, the uterus looks like this. On the left is the cervix, and on the right the body of the uterus. Above the baby is the placenta, or afterbirth. Practise your drills every day, and particularly those in the two previous sections, preferably with another person helping you. The uterus is mostly supporting the weight of the baby in its bag of fluid, as well as the weight of the placenta. During the last few weeks of pregnancy, the uterus may make several 'trial runs' for labour. You will feel gentle but firm tightening around your 'bulge', and it's a good idea to breathe through it for practice and experience. Just lean against the sink, using your hands for support, or slump in a chair and breathe in level A.

2 Here the cervix, or narrow end of the uterus, is being pulled up in preparation for opening, but is not open yet. The contractions you feel will be stronger, and more regular than the 'trial run', but still quite gentle. Contractions should be breathed through if you happen to be awake, otherwise get plenty of rest and sleep. Don't go on long journeys, and stay at home apart from a short walk or a little shopping. Contractions will usually be gentle enough to handle with level A or level B breathing.

Some tips:

- Don't take a big gulp of air during controlled breathing – your chest muscles are contracted. Just blow out gently until you feel yourself going loose inside your bra, then carry on with controlled breathing.

- If you feel 'trembly' make all your breathing more pronounced, and make sure that the out breath is firmer than the in breath.

- If your feet feel cold, wear woolly socks: all the body energy is being concentrated round the uterus, and blood circulation to your feet is neglected.

- Each labour is different, and what you read here and elsewhere about length of labour and contractions can only be guidelines. Suit your actions to the particular behaviour of your body.

Continued overleaf

3 Now the uterus has started to open the cervix almost to its full extent. The baby's head is at the entrance to the birth canal. The contractions will be strong and frequent, often 1½ to 2 minutes long, with only a minute's rest in between. You will either be in hospital or on your way there. Lay in the basic position as you did in your drill, and handle each contraction. You will probably need all four levels of controlled breathing, and the longest part will be the strongest part of the contraction, needing breathing level D – your song and light tapping routine. Rest between contractions, take a sip of water if you feel dry and *be patient.*

4 If you feel that your strongest sensations during the contraction of the uterus are in your lower back, lay in the position shown here.

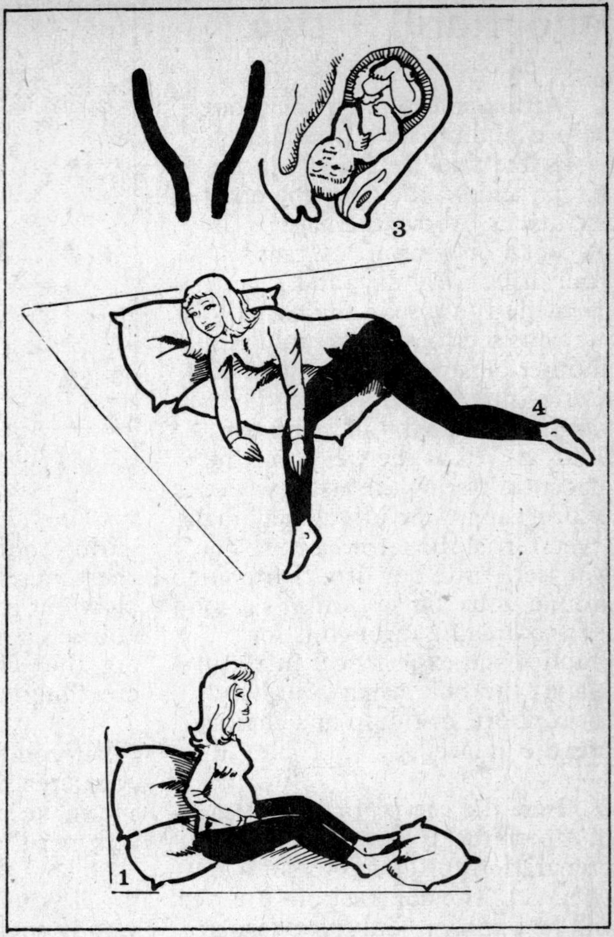

two ways at once

Until now you have made the responses to the signals from the uterus and therefore you have stayed 'on top', in control. Now there will be a sudden change. You will feel, or rather most women do, the strong pull of the muscles still opening the cervix and also the first sensations of muscle-push which is a sign that the uterus is preparing for the 'pushing' or second stage of labour. However strong the pushing-feeling is, *you must not join in yet.* You must wait with your pushing-efforts until you are told to push by the doctor or nurse.

1 Choose this, or the following position, whichever you find most comfortable. Here you sit up straight, as if you were sitting on a rather wide see-saw. Push your bottom well backwards against your pillows. Upper part of the back should be free. Bend your

knees loosely and rest legs lightly against a pillow in front of them.

2 This position is very similar to the one described for the situation of having backache during labour. But your under-arm should be pulled forward, so that the hand is lying next to your face.

The controlled breathing drill to go with this part of labour is a bit tricky until you have learnt the knack, so it needs as much practice as the other drills for labour. The contraction will be very powerful and will rise to its height very quickly; so one breath in level A, two or three breaths in level B and a few seconds in level C and you will feel a muddled, strong sensation when you immediately let your upper body slump forward and let the air in your chest escape. Then sit up and mime the count of '1–2, 1–2,' letting your breathing come naturally. Then again slump and let the air out and go back to '1–2, 1–2,' mime repeat again and again until the contraction feels weaker and you can stay on top with ordinary controlled breathing Level C, and so on down through the levels until the contraction has gone.

With luck you'll have a few moments to rest and then the uterus will start once more and you go with it. Don't fall into the error of panting wildly during the height of these contractions – you will 'overbreathe' and make yourself dizzy, which is not very good for

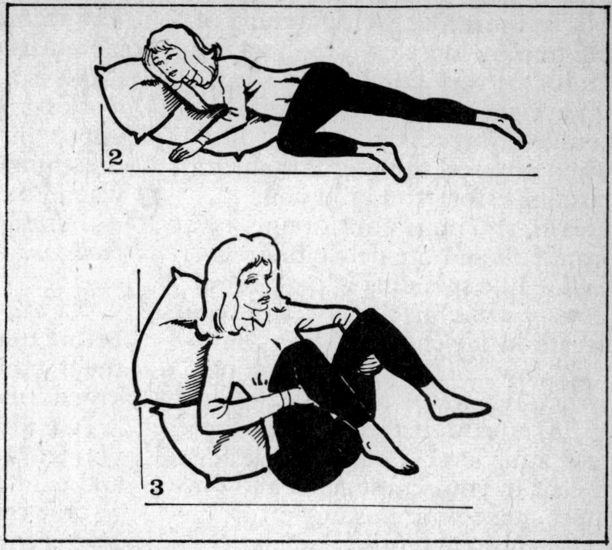

the baby either. This part of labour may last only about 20 minutes, but it may go on for much longer. Try to remember, though, that quite soon you'll be told *'You can push now.*

3 The position you will be asked to get into is usually as shown here. Between contractions you can rest with your legs lying comfortably in front of you. But when each contraction begins, grab your thighs as in the diagram (practise this as part of your labour-drill) and make sure that you bend as though *trying to touch your knees with your nose*. Don't try to bring your knees up as far as you can – this would tighten the muscles around the outlet from your body. When you feel the contraction beginning it

Continued overleaf

will feel just like the tightening of the tummy-muscles – by now this should be very familiar. So use these eight to 10 seconds to take a couple of breaths in level A. But when you feel the uterus make its pushing effort you hold your breath, and push your tummy away from you and the pelvic floor as well – like spending a 'big penny' (lots of urine) in a hurry. Hold your breath in the chest and put your chin down for your best pushing effort. When you must breathe in again, release the held breath and take a big level A breath in, hold the air in your chest again and once more make your pushing-effort.

When you are sure that the uterus is not pushing any more, you stop too, *lie back gently and breathe in level C* until you can rest normally. Don't fling yourself back, and avoid unnecessary movements so that you don't let the baby's head slide backwards in the vagina more than is absolutely essential. For the next contraction which will begin a few minutes later, off you go again, repeating the same drill.

The second, or delivery, stage of labour usually lasts about one hour if this is a first baby and you will be working really hard. It is very important to practise the breathing/hold breath/push drill when you practise all the other labour drills, but during practice *push only with your tummy muscles, not your pelvic floor.*

Right at the end, a few moments before your baby is actually born, the doctor or nurse will suddenly say, during a pushing-contraction, 'STOP PUSHING!' Immediately you let the air out of your chest and pant gently to allow the uterus to urge the baby's head out of your body gently. Your added effort could make this too fast and cause damage to your pelvic floor. The rest of the baby's body will slide out almost without your noticing and then you will meet him for the first time, perhaps even be allowed to hold him in your arms.

Usually the afterbirth, or placenta, is released by the uterus a few minutes later, needing just a little pushing effort from you.

the unusual labour

The drills described above are intended to show what usually happens when women give birth. There are labours where, for medical reasons particular to an individual woman, the labour is different in some ways but not in others. The doctor may decide to start your labour in hospital with drugs or he may give you medicines by injection to hurry labour along; perhaps during the delivery of your baby it may be that your efforts and those of the uterus are not strong enough to push the baby out of your body without help from the doctor.

All these and many other things may make it different from the description I have given. However, what you know and the ways in which you have taught yourself to help yourself to stay in control must be of use to you, even if you can't make it all the way. Remember that whatever you or the doctor or nurse can do to help will make the experience for you and your baby more satisfactory. Your understanding of how to stay with your body's efforts can only be of value.

post-natal exercises

by Mai Bryson

The first half of the exercises are non-weight bearing and should be done during the 14 days following the birth (with the consent of your doctor).

The first day do exercises 1 and 2.

The second day add 3 and 4.

The third day add 5 and 6.

The fourth day add 7 and 8.

Continue with these 8 exercises for 14 days.

The number of repetitions should be increased each day according to how strong you are feeling.

Do not forget to do the breathing exercise before starting the programme, in the middle and at the end of the routine.

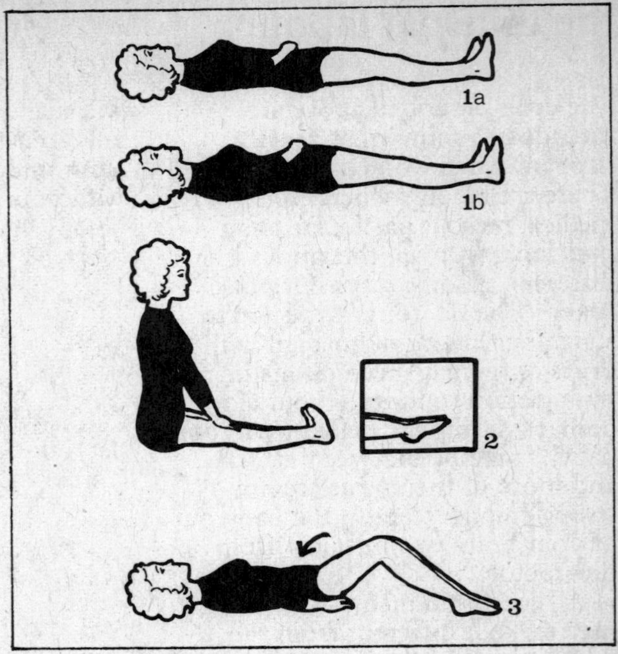

improving circulation

1a and b With hands on abdomen breathe in deeply allowing tummy to relax then pull in tummy and breathe out. Repeat 4 times.

strengthening legs

2 Sitting on a bed with hands on thighs, bend feet up and down to full extent. Then rotate your ankles, first in one direction then the other. Repeat each exercise 10 times.

strengthening abdomen

3 Lie on your back with knees bent and feet resting on bed. Tighten your buttocks and press the middle of your back down on bed. Relax. Repeat 6 times.

strengthening waist muscles – one

4a Lie down, with right knee bent and left leg straight. Slide the heel of the left leg as far down as possible. Then, still keeping the left leg straight, slide the heel up as far as possible.

4b Repeat the exercise, but this time with the left knee bent and the right leg straight.

4c Now slide the bent right knee up and down . . .

4d . . . and then slide the bent left knee up and down.

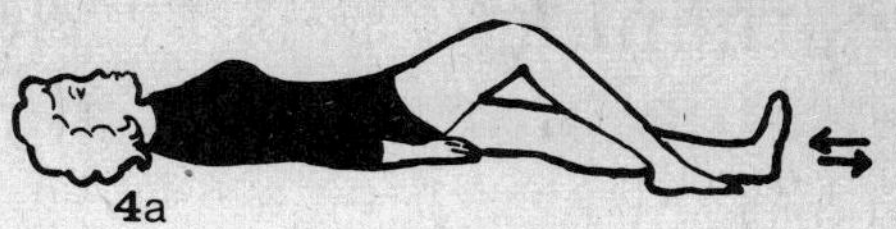

4a

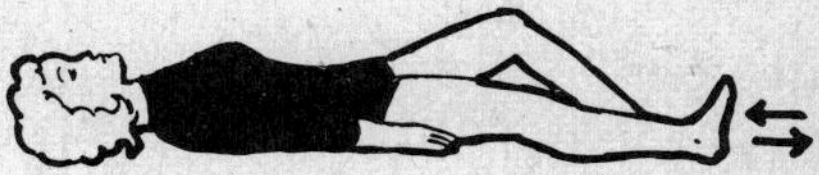

4b

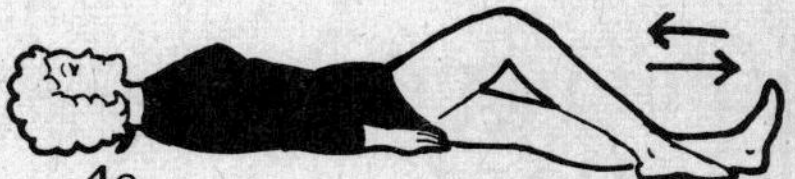

4c

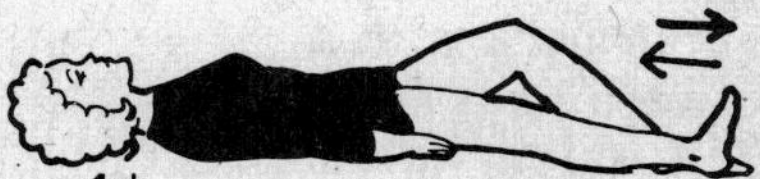

4d

strengthening waist muscles – two

5a Lie on your back, with your knees bent and legs supported only by toes. Keep the knees together and the shoulders flat.

5b Let the closed legs fall gently to the right until they are resting on the floor, with the left hip raised and the waist twisted.

Return knees to original position and repeat exercise, but this time falling to the left. Do exercise six times in each direction.

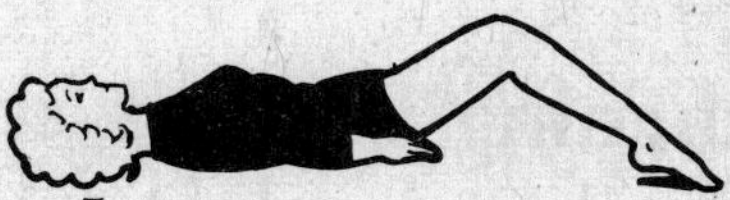

5a

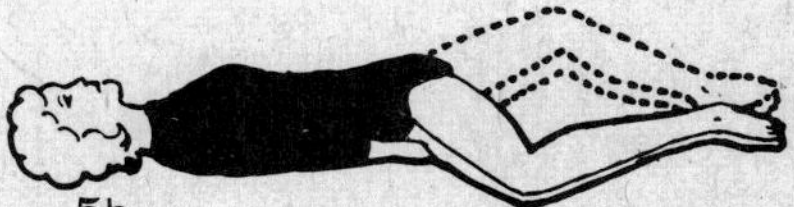

5b

strengthening abdominal muscles

6a Lie on your back.

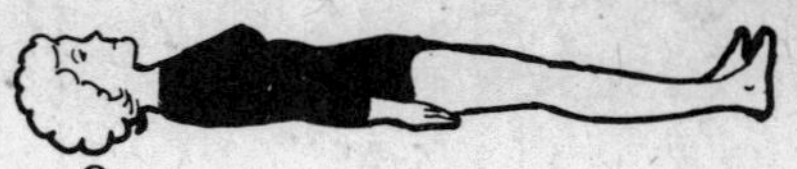

6a

6b Raise your head and shoulders, and hold position for five seconds before relaxing.

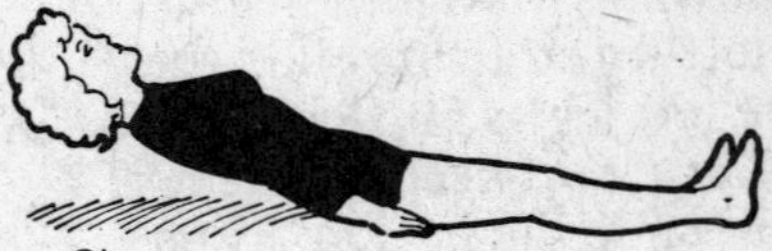

6b

strengthening muscles of pelvic floor

7 Lie on your back with a cushion between your knees. Squeeze the cushion, holding tight for five seconds before relaxing. Do exercise six times.

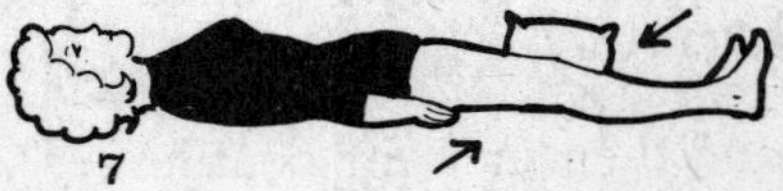

7

8 Do the same exercise as above, but bend the knees upwards. Do exercise six times.

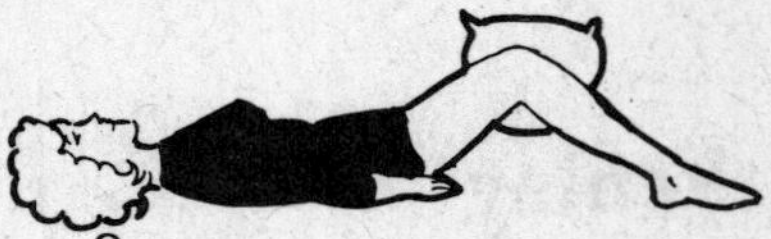

8

strengthening abdominal and pelvic floor muscles

9a Lie on your back with cushion between knees. Breathe in and raise your body on your shoulders. Hold the position for five seconds . . .

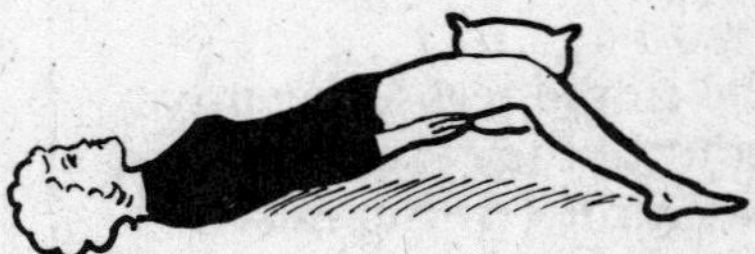

9a

9b . . . then relax to floor, breathing out. Do exercise six times.

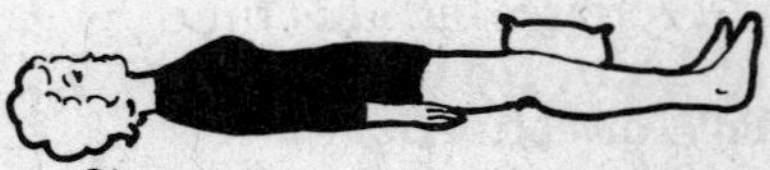

9b

circulation in the breasts

10a Sit on chair with fingertips touching your shoulders.

10b Make circles with your elbows fairly quickly, 10 times each way. Do exercise three times.

abdominal circulation and constipation

11a Lie on your back, breathe in and raise the right leg . . .

11b . . . as far up on the chest as possible. Press it gently on abdomen, then stretch out leg straight, breathing out at the same time.

11c Now breathe in and raise the left leg . . .

11d . . . as far up on the chest as possible. Stretch the leg out straight, breathing out at the same time. Do the exercise six times with each leg.

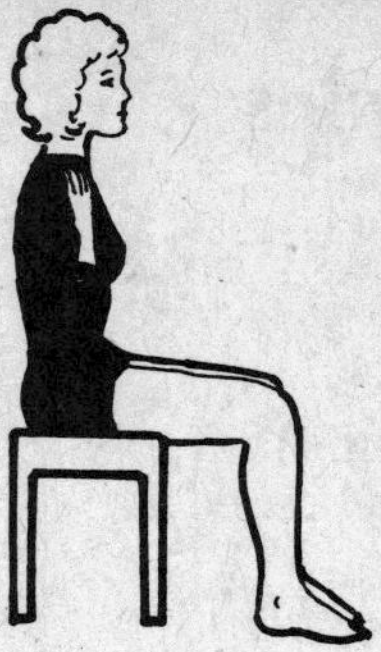
10a

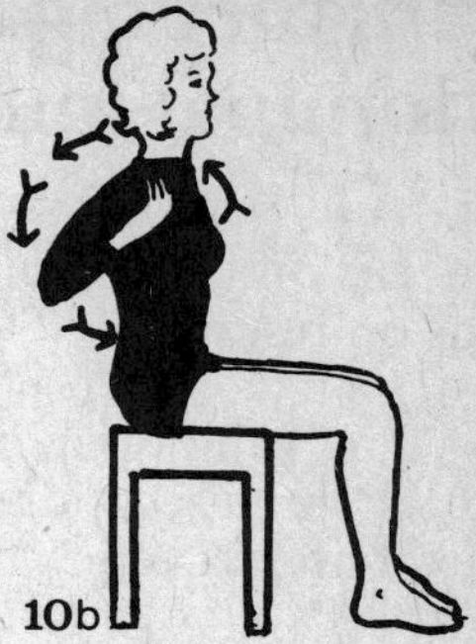
10b

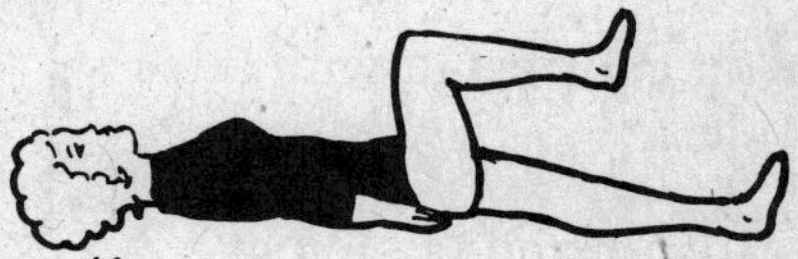
11a

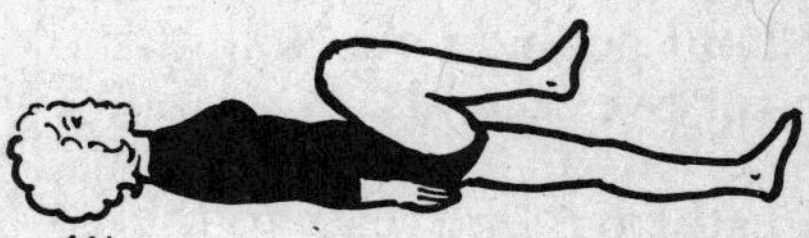
11b

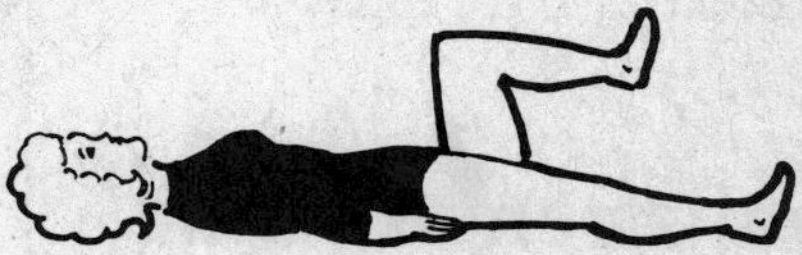
11c

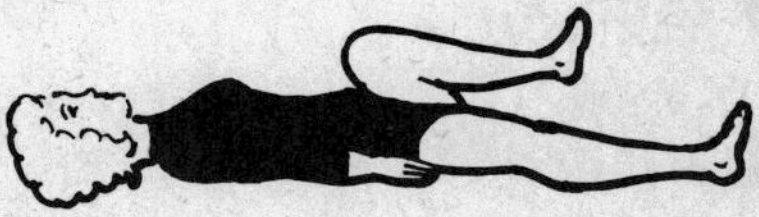
11d

strengthening abdominal muscles

12a Lie on your front, with both hands on tummy.

12b Pull tummy up from floor, hold for three seconds and relax. Do exercise six times.

strengthening back muscles

13a Lie on your front, with arms by your sides.

13b Breathe in and raise your head and shoulders, with your arms stretched out behind you. Hold this position for five seconds.

13c Breathe out and relax to the floor. Do exercise six times.

general strengthening exercises

14a Kneel down on all fours.

14b Breathe in and arch your back like a cat. Hold this position for five seconds, then relax to your original position, breathing out. Do the exercise six times.

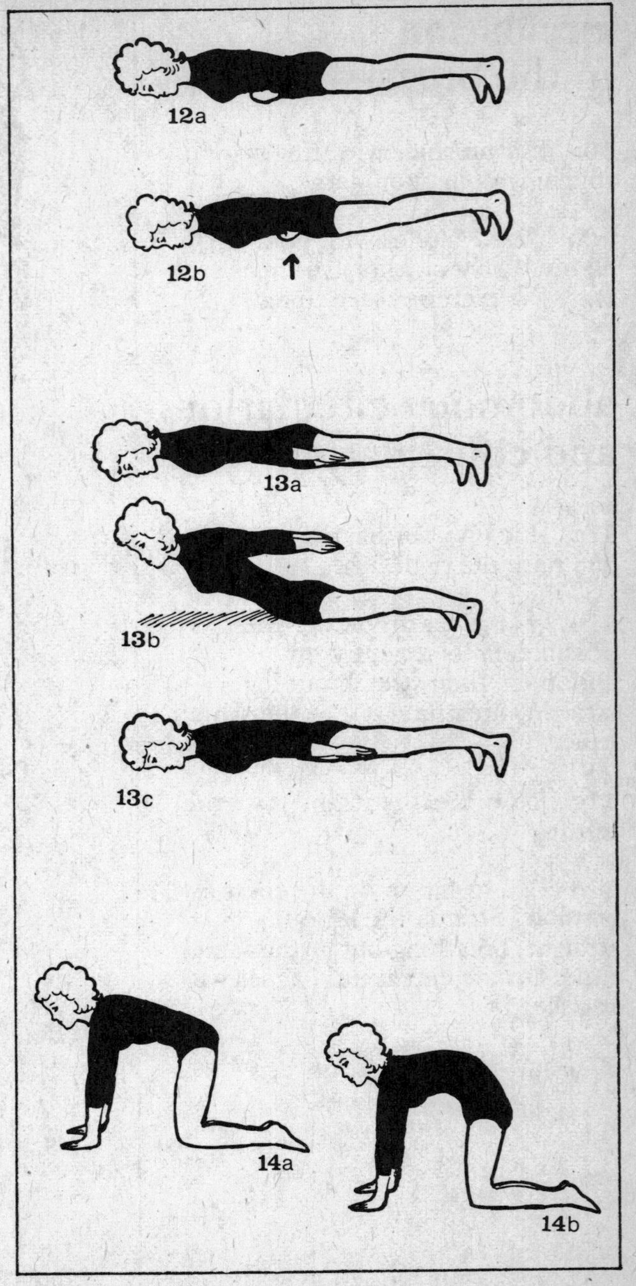

stronger exercise for waist

This is similar to exercise 4, but is done in the standing position.

15a Pull your right leg up, making it short, and hold the position for five seconds before returning the foot to the floor.

15b Repeat the action with the left leg. Do exercise six times with each leg.

strengthening and trimming waist

16a Stand with the left hand on the waist and the right hand by your side.

16b Bend your body to the right in three dipping movements, so that your right hand goes farther down your right leg every time.
Return to standing position, and repeat the exercise, this time dipping the left arm down the left leg. Do the exercise six times for each leg.

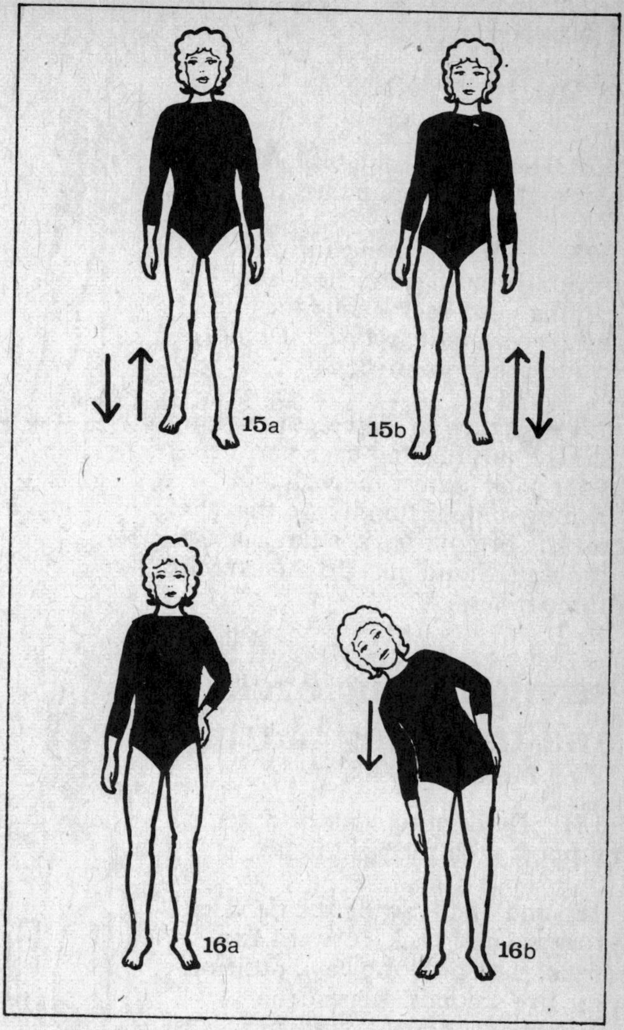

flattening a hollow back

17a Stand against a wall, with your feet about six inches forward.

17b Gradually bend forward, tucking your head in first, and curling your back, while the arms hang down quite relaxed. Do not try to touch your toes.

17c Return to the erect position slowly, pushing out each part of your back against the wall and pulling in your tummy, so that the middle of your back is flat against the wall. Stand tall. Do the exercise three times.

strengthening back and trimming buttocks

18a Hold on to chair or other support with the right hand.

18b and 18c Swing the right leg forward and back, forward and back, then hold the back position for five seconds. Repeat the exercise four times. Now turn round and grip the chair with the left hand, and swing the left leg, with a five second hold on the back swing. Do this four times.

By the end of one month or six weeks, exercises like cycling, running on the spot with knee

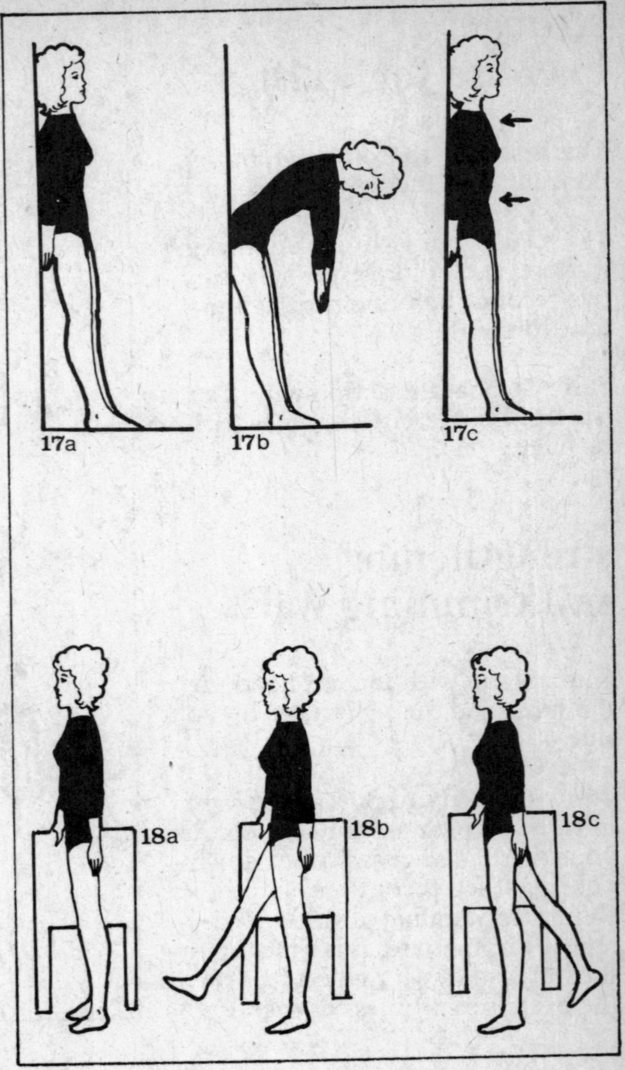

raising, and more general exercises can be done. Be careful not to lift heavy weights. Bend your knees, not your back when lifting your baby.